THE FAST REVOLUTION

TOP 100

taste.COM.AU

THE FAST REVOLUTION

THE BEST OF THE BEST RECIPES FROM AUSTRALIA'S #1 FOOD SITE

HarperCollinsPublishers

CONTENTS

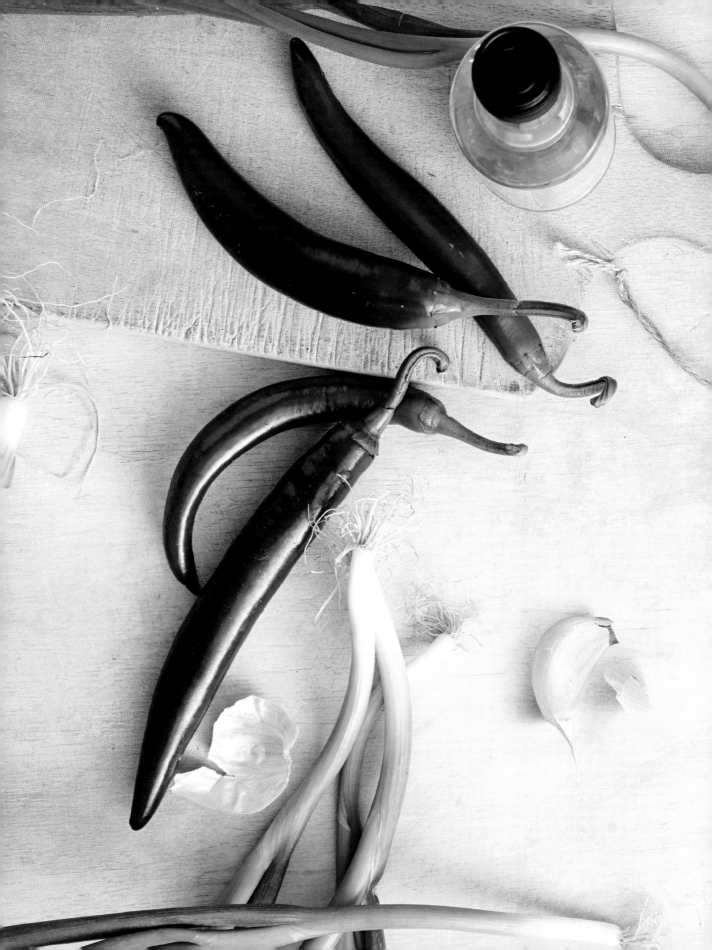

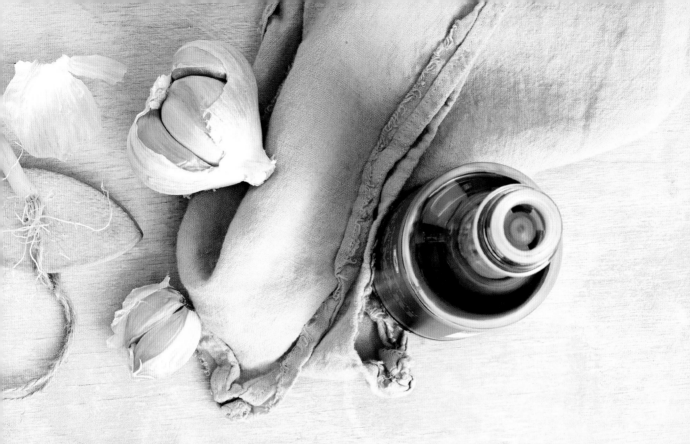

HELLO!

If you're reading this book, like me, you're probably intrigued by the idea of intermittent fasting. And why wouldn't you be? It's not often something with so many potential health benefits comes along – from delayed ageing, to reduced risk of a huge range of chronic diseases such as cancer, diabetes and heart disease.

Problem is, straight old calorie restriction is not much fun, especially for food lovers. Who really wants to spend their days counting calories? Plus, while there's a lot of information out there about the why of intermittent fasting, there's much less about

how to actually do it, let alone quick and easy ideas for true foodies.

With *The Fast Revolution*, intermittent fasting meets real life. This is your perfect planner for fasting and non-fasting days alike, expertly curated by taste.com.au's food and nutrition teams. Best of all, *The Fast Revolution* is designed for everyone. No matter who you are, no matter your size, gender, exercise level or your dietary preferences.

And you certainly won't go hungry! The dishes in *The Fast Revolution* may be low in calories but they truly satisfy, with big flavour,

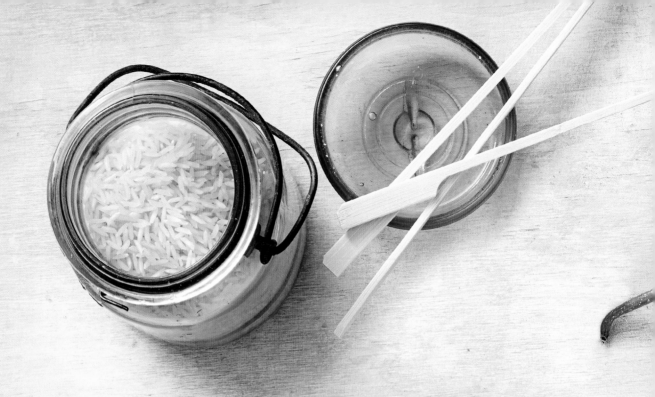

My personal favourite feature is the truly innovative approach to meal plans.

lots of hearty goodness and loads of fresh seasonal ingredients.

Snacks are included too. In fact, they're an essential part of the formula to keep you satisfied. We want *The Fast Revolution* to help you enjoy life, not deny life's pleasures. Sure, you'll probably be dialling down portion sizes for high-calorie treats, but we're not into 'banned' lists (that's why we've included a calorie counter for non-diet treats too).

The recipes are also easy to adapt for non-fasting days – just follow the tips for twisting the recipe to make it more substantial, or making it for non-fasting

family members. Plus, we've included at-a-glance key guides to vegan, vegetarian, and gluten-free recipes, as well as make-ahead and freezable options.

My personal favourite feature is the truly innovative approach to meal plans. This is something I've been wanting for such a long time. Finally, I have limitless daily meal plan options at my fingertips, with all the guides, tools, tips and tricks to get on track – and stay on track. No more guesswork.

As with every taste.com.au recipe, all the ingredients are at your local supermarket to make planning and cooking affordable and

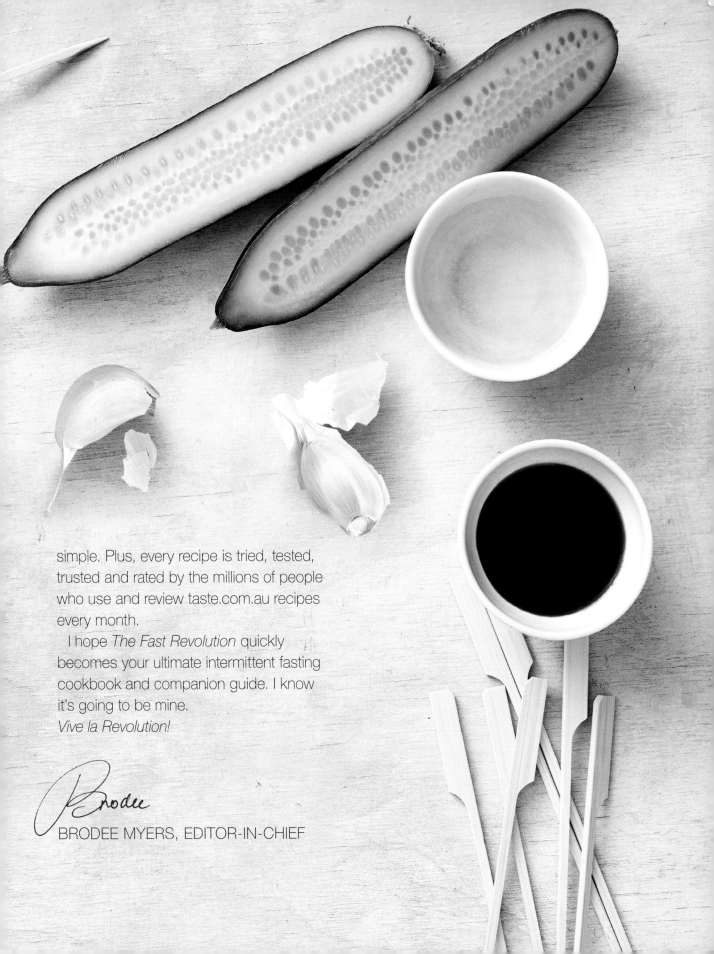

simple. Plus, every recipe is tried, tested, trusted and rated by the millions of people who use and review taste.com.au recipes every month.

I hope *The Fast Revolution* quickly becomes your ultimate intermittent fasting cookbook and companion guide. I know it's going to be mine.

Vive la Revolution!

BRODEE MYERS, EDITOR-IN-CHIEF

HOW TO USE
THE FAST REVOLUTION

Welcome to taste.com.au's *The Fast Revolution*, with all the recipes, tools, tips and guides you need to achieve your health and weight-loss goals.

AMAZING FEATURES

Full prep & cooking times

Complete nutritional information

5-star recipe ratings

At-a-glance calorie counter

Reviews from home cooks

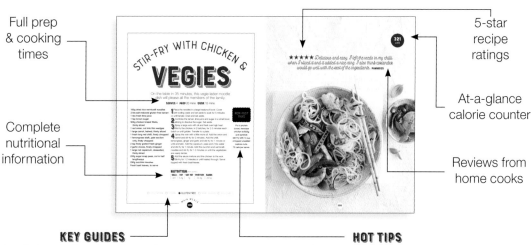

KEY GUIDES
Highlighted dots indicating gluten-free, vegan, vegetarian, make-ahead and freezable meals

HOT TIPS
Helpful hints, including easy twists for non-fasting days

DO IT YOUR WAY

All the recipes are divided into three separate calorie-counted sections: Main Meals, Light Meals and Snacks. No more boring calorie counting!

MAIN MEALS
500 CALORIES

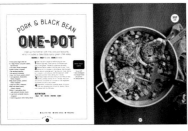

Hearty yet healthy, our main meals section has inspiring recipes that are all 500 calories or less.

LIGHT MEALS
250 CALORIES

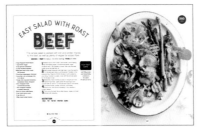

The carefully curated collection of light meals are perfect for keeping your fasting days on track.

SNACKS
125 CALORIES

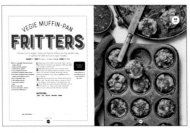

This chapter proves you don't need to give up snacks! Choose from sweet and savoury options.

MIX & MATCH GUIDES

Here's your daily and weekly meal planner where you can see every meal at a glance, with key guides, calorie count and page number listed on each recipe.

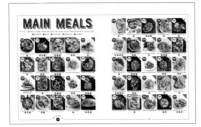

Choose which main meals you're having based on dietary preferences and discover your options for make-ahead and freezable meals.

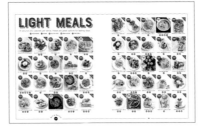

Plan your fasting days simply and quickly by choosing your favourite lighter meal options that are still delicious and filling.

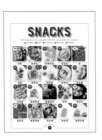

Did someone say snacks? Prevent hunger, satisfy any sweet cravings and supplement your healthy eating plan with these delicious snack options.

HANDY GUIDES

To help keep you on track with your healthy eating goals,
we've included a wealth of other handy features in *The Fast Revolution*.

CALORIE CHART

The Fast Revolution is about real life,
so here's your go-to calorie counter for
all those extras. There's fruit and veg,
plus nibbles and drinks – even wine!

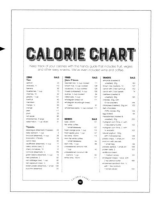

FRESH SNACKS IN SEASON

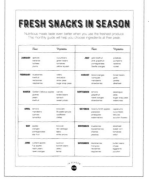

Fruit and veg are the cornerstone of any
healthy meal plan. Nothing beats fresh food
in season at the peak of nutrients – and value
too! Use this month-by-month guide, plus
help your budget, because if it's in season, it's
usually cheaper. Use our guide to stay savvy.

EASY MEAL PLANS

Here's your formula for building your daily
meal plans. Just use the sample guides
from taste.com.au nutrition editor Chrissy
Freer, then choose your meals from the
Mix & Match guides. Or invent your own
module, it's completely up to you!

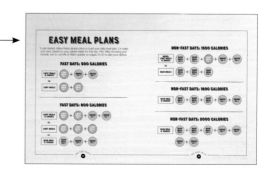

INDEXES

INDEX BY OCCASION

Discover your favourite meals by occasion, whether it's breakfast, lunch, dinner, snacks or sweets.

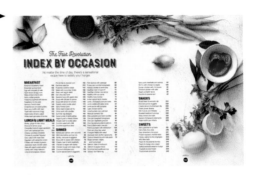

INDEX BY MEAL TYPE

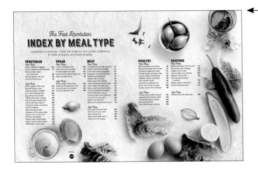

This quick finder helps you find all your vegan and vegetarian options, and also provides listings for meat, poultry and seafood.

INDEX BY KEY GUIDE

This index sorts the recipes according to special criteria, such as gluten-free, vegan, vegetarian as well as being freezer-friendly and make-ahead.

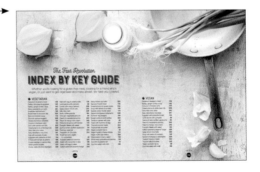

THE TASTE.COM.AU GUARANTEE

All taste.com.au recipes are triple-tested, rated and reviewed by Aussie cooks just like you. Plus, every ingredient is as close as your local supermarket.

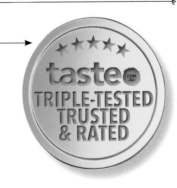

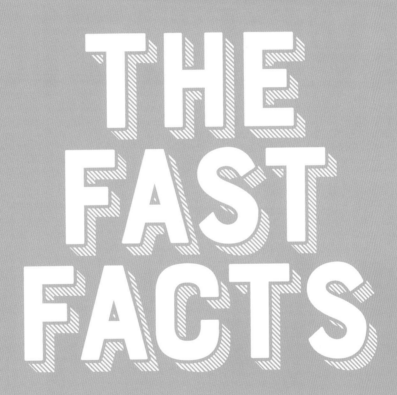

THE FAST FACTS

ALL YOU NEED TO KNOW ABOUT INTERMITTENT
FASTING, INCLUDING YOUR EASY MEAL PLANS.

ALL ABOUT THE FAST REVOLUTION

Taste.com.au's nutrition editor Chrissy Freer explains what intermittent fasting means and how it can help you lose weight – and keep it off.

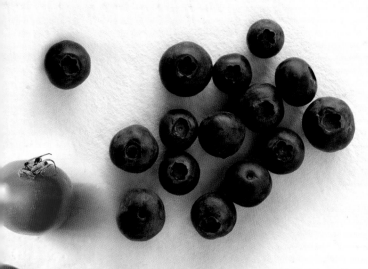

There's a lot of talk about intermittent fasting these days. With two out of every three Australian adults now overweight or obese, and diseases such as type 2 diabetes becoming serious health issues, strategies to successfully lose and manage weight have never been so important. Alternating periods of fasting with normal eating has certainly been shown to be a powerful tool for improving overall health.

As a nutritionist, what I like about intermittent fasting as a weight-loss strategy is that it's often much more sustainable than simply cutting calories day in, day out. Many people find the daily grind of calorie counting too difficult. With intermittent fasting you effectively compress your low-calorie eating to certain days or certain hours per day – which is often much easier and more realistic. For example, rather than every day of the week being a 'diet day', you have, say, two diet days per week. And instead of cutting out a little each day, you cut a lot more calories on those two days. This means you can enjoy your usual eating pattern for the rest of the week.

Many studies have shown that this is an effective method of dieting for people. Let's take a look at the evidence and what the science says.

> 66 *There are several variations of intermittent fasting, differing in length and frequency of the fast cycle, so you can tailor a plan to suit your individual needs and lifestyle.* 99

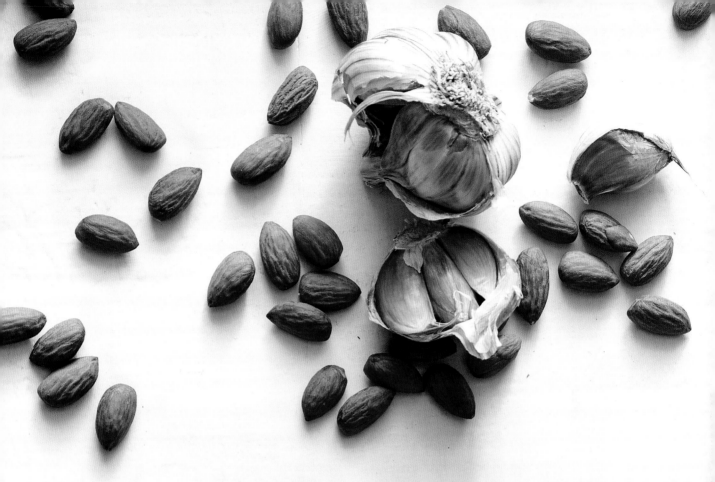

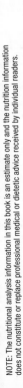

THE SCIENCE

Because it's so flexible, for many, intermittent fasting doesn't seem as difficult as traditional weight-loss methods, which is why you are more likely to lose the weight you want.

Intermittent fasting works in a similar way to traditional diets. Typically, most diets recommend reducing daily calories by about 500-1000 calories. Generally speaking, cutting 500 calories each day reduces your weight by half a kilo per week.

One of our aims with *The Fast Revolution* is to show you how to achieve the same result by reducing your total *weekly* calories. This results in the same impressive weight-loss benefits, and you can even change how many fasting days you choose per week to achieve faster or slower results.

The science of intermittent fasting, however, goes way beyond just calorie cutting for weight loss. Scientific evidence suggests that intermittent fasting may improve insulin sensitivity and glucose levels, lower blood pressure, and reduce body fat and therefore inflammation. It's also been shown to be effective at reducing ectopic fat.

This unhealthy fat around organs, such as liver, heart and pancreas, is associated with type 2 diabetes. And, if you fast for 12 hours or more, such as with time-restricted fasting, the body can switch to a ketogenic metabolic mode, using ketone bodies (derived from fat) and free fatty acids as energy sources during the fasting period.

Time-restricted eating can also positively influence circadian rhythms, our bodies' natural 24-hour cycle. It's believed that aspects of cell repair and rejuvenation are also associated with periods of fasting. The fasting appears to help the body reset, which explains why intermittent fasting may be important for optimising health and longevity.

However, it's important to note that fasting diets are not appropriate for everyone and you should seek medical advice before starting a fasting plan. In particular, they should not be used for children, the elderly or those who are under the healthy weight range. Diabetics should also seek medical advice before undertaking fasting plans.

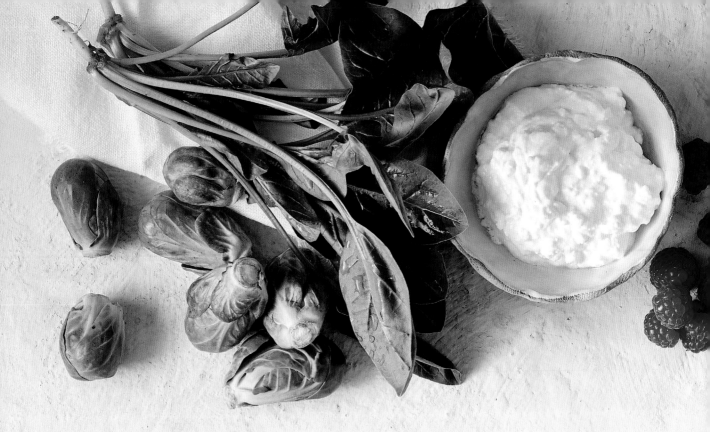

WHAT TYPE OF FASTING IS RIGHT FOR YOU?

5:2 Intermittent fasting

One of the most popular intermittent fasting variations is the 5:2 intermittent fasting plan championed by Dr Michael Mosley and Mimi Spencer in his 2013 book, *The Fast Diet* (Short Books). For this version, fasting days are very light in calories. In fact, fasting day calories are cut to 500 calories per day (women) or 600 calories (men). This is about one-quarter of the recommended daily intake to maintain weight. As the name suggests, you fast on just two days per week, then for five days a week you eat either a normal diet, which is about 1800-2000 calories for adult women and 1900-2400 calories for adult men, or a lighter version of a normal day (around 1500 calories per day).

The Mosley system means you choose which days you want to fast – to fit in with your lifestyle choices and schedule. For example, if you know you have a special dinner planned, move your fasting day to accommodate.

Typically, weekdays make easier fasting days, as eating tends to be more structured and you are in routine, but the choice is yours. Some people break up the two days, others prefer to fast two days consecutively. Some find it's easier to get the fasting done on Monday and Tuesday, leaving the rest of the week to eat normally.

It is also important to note that while you do not need to calorie count on non-fasting days, if you want to lose weight, you shouldn't over-compensate by eating badly. You still need to cut calories over the course of the week, which means over-indulging on non-fasting days can derail your good work. Snacking on lower-calorie foods, such as vegie sticks and fresh berries, is a great way to avoid hunger on fasting days. See our calorie chart on page 31 for ideas. And, importantly, once you lose those extra kilos and want to maintain your new healthy weight, the 5:2 plan can be a great way to stay on track for the future.

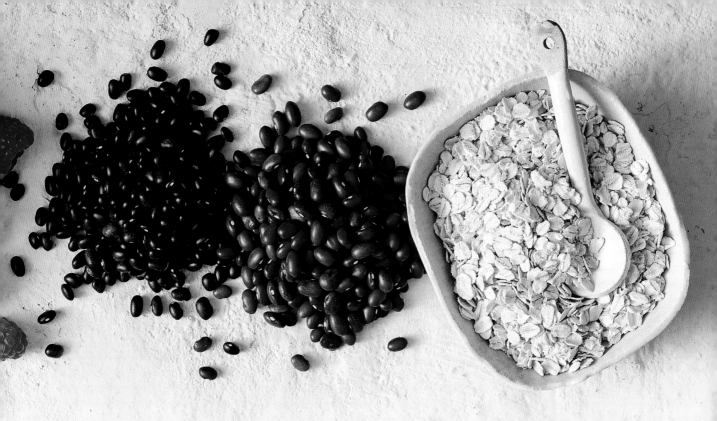

Time-restricted eating

Another popular form of intermittent fasting is known as time-restricted eating. This approach involves stretching out the time of your usual overnight fast (which is when you sleep). This type of fasting plan is usually implemented every day. A common version involves a 16-hour fast, leaving an eight-hour eating period each day. For example, you may have your last meal at 7pm, then fast overnight and not eat again until 11am the next morning. Fasting periods of 12 hours and 10 hours can also be beneficial.

Time-restricted eating does not typically require calorie counting. However, by reducing eating to only eight hours per day, a natural reduction in calories often occurs. Worried that you will overeat at lunch as a consequence? Evidence suggests that this is not the case.

If you are someone who does not like to skip breakfast, try eating your dinner earlier. Generally speaking, intermittent fasting is a great way to stop late-night snacking, which often results in unwanted extra calories. (Who hasn't been tempted by the fridge in the late evening?) And it's not just about weight loss. According to scientific studies, time-restricted eating is also associated with improvements in several health-related biomarkers, such as insulin sensitivity and inflammation, as well as longevity and wellbeing. It can be a wonderful tool for weight maintenance and improving your overall health.

800 calorie intermittent fasting

Again, the leading proponent of this approach is Dr Mosley in his 2018 book, *The Fast 800* (Simon & Schuster), where he updated the 5:2 approach, based on science that shows 800 calories is effective. This approach to fasting incorporates both 5:2 and time-restricted eating, and involves reducing calorie intake to 800 calories per day, as well as incorporating overnight fasts of 12 hours or more (say from 7pm until 7am the next morning).

In contrast to 5:2, *The Fast 800* plan starts with 800 calories every day for two weeks, up to a maximum of 12 weeks. You then transition to a 5:2 style, with 800 calories for at least two days per week. For a gentler version, or for weight maintenance, start on 800 calories for two days per week. Men may wish to add an extra snack or light meal to increase their intake to around 1000 calories per day for this protocol.

The Fast 800 adopts a Mediterranean-style diet on fasting and non-fasting days. Acclaimed by nutritionists for healthy eating, heart health and preventing diabetes, the Mediterranean diet is linked to reducing the risk of chronic disease, chronic inflammation and promoting wellbeing. It involves eating lots of fresh fruit, vegies and legumes, moderate serves of lean protein (especially fish, lean chicken and eggs) and wholegrains with small serves of good fats, such as extra virgin olive oil, nuts, seeds and avocados. You will find most of the recipes in *The Fast Revolution* also take this Mediterranean-style approach.

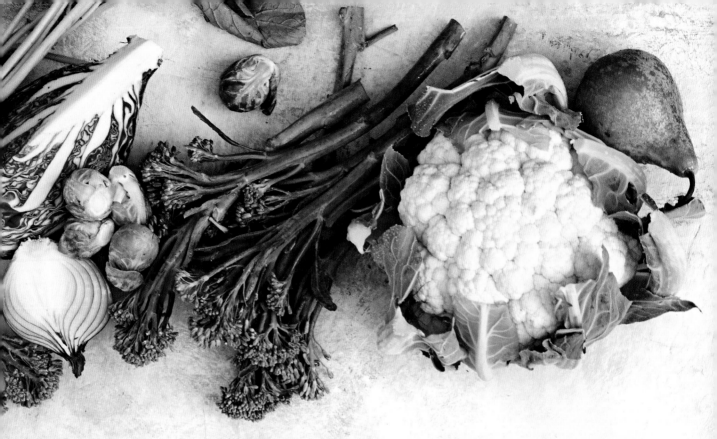

HOW TO START

No matter which variant of intermittent fasting you feel is right for you, *The Fast Revolution* has the tools to make it easy and achievable. We've divided the recipes into three handy sections: main meals; light meals; and snacks. With these three sections you can easily build your daily meal plan.

Main meals

These 500 calorie or less recipes are ideal for both fasting and non-fasting days. They also help with maintenance once you reach your goal weight. To make it even more user-friendly, we've included timesaving tips, such as make-ahead tags and freezable recipes. *See pages 32-123.*

Light meals

Perfect for fasting days, these recipes of around 250 calories are also a great option when you simply want a leaner choice for breakfast, lunch or dinner. *See pages 124-215.*

Snacks

These healthy snacks of less than 125 calories are a critical part of successful intermittent fasting, helping you maintain energy levels and stave off hunger. *See pages 216-242.*

Calorie counter

It's not all about recipes. Use our handy calorie counter on page 31 to track your favourite foods and snacks.

Special diets & food preferences

Each recipe contains at-a-glance guides to special dietary needs and preferences such as gluten free, vegetarian and vegan, as well as full nutritional information.

Tips & twists for non-fasting days

Many recipes include tips to twist recipes for non-fasting days, making recipes a little more substantial and filling.

Weight maintenance requirements

Want to maintain your weight? General targets are about 1800-2000 calories a day for adult women and 1900-2400 calories for adult men, depending on age. These figures are only averages and actual energy needs will vary dependent upon activity levels, body composition, health, weight and height. For example, some women may find they need to keep to 1700 calories per day, while someone who is very active can eat more than the recommended intake.

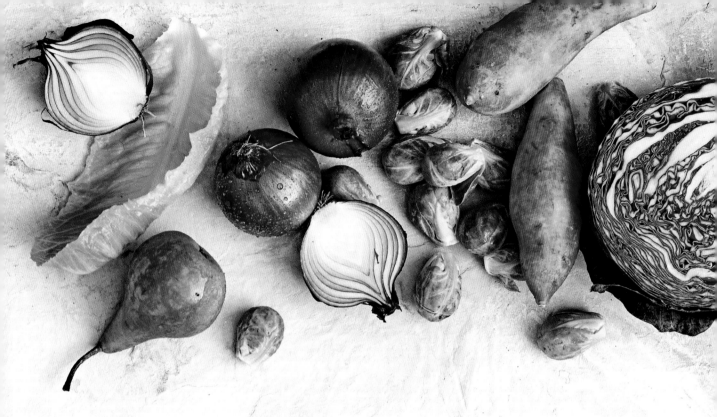

HOW TO ADD FLAVOUR WITHOUT CALORIES

Dried spices & herbs

Spice up lean cuts of meat, such as chicken breast, pork loin steaks, lamb cutlets or lean beef, with a dry spice rub before grilling, or sprinkle over vegetables before roasting. Some great zero-calorie combinations include:
● ground cumin, paprika, ground coriander
● crushed fennel seeds, lemon zest, chopped rosemary
● smoked paprika, ground cumin, pinch of ground cinnamon
● dried chilli flakes, paprika, lemon zest, dried oregano

Fresh herbs & spices

● Add fresh herbs and chilli to salads for instant flavour and freshness, or to low-cal salad dressings for a flavour boost.
● Try tossing them through stir-fries at the very end of cooking or sprinkle fresh herbs over soups, stews and curries to serve.
● Fresh ginger, garlic and lemongrass add punch to stir-fries, Asian salads, soups and dressings.

Salad dressings

When making salad dressings, use orange, lemon or lime juice as the base, rather than olive oil. Add no more than 1 tsp olive oil per serve. Natural yoghurt is also a great option for a low-fat creamy dressing.

Condiments

● Limit your intake of sugar-laden sauces, such as plum sauce, sweet chilli, hoisin, oyster sauce, and high-fat dressings, such as mayonnaise, aïoli, ranch and satay sauce. Instead, opt for wholegrain and Dijon mustard, or hot chilli sauce (only use a little).
● Homemade apple sauce or no-added-sugar apple puree are also a good choice, while tzatziki is great in wraps or serve it with grilled meats.
● For stir-fries and Asian salad dressings, rice wine vinegar, Chinese rice wine, soy sauce and fish sauce are relatively low cal but can be high in sodium, so moderation is key.

Chrissy Freer is a qualified nutritionist (B App Sc Nut, Grad Dip Human Nut), health author and recipe developer with more than 20 years industry experience. She is a member of the Nutrition Society of Australia.

EASY MEAL PLANS

To get started, follow these simple plans to build your daily meal plan. Or make your own, based on your calorie intake for that day. Hint: After choosing your module, turn to our Mix & Match guides on pages 24-30 to plan your dishes.

FAST DAYS: 500 CALORIES

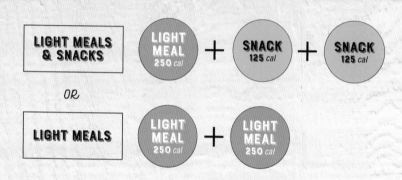

LIGHT MEALS & SNACKS
LIGHT MEAL 250 cal + SNACK 125 cal + SNACK 125 cal

OR

LIGHT MEALS
LIGHT MEAL 250 cal + LIGHT MEAL 250 cal

FAST DAYS: 800 CALORIES

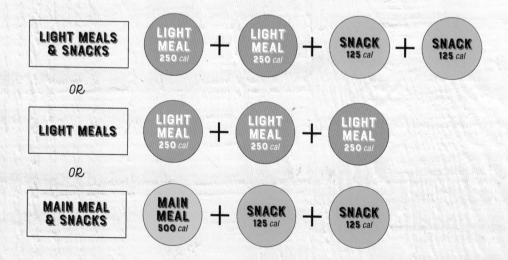

LIGHT MEALS & SNACKS
LIGHT MEAL 250 cal + LIGHT MEAL 250 cal + SNACK 125 cal + SNACK 125 cal

OR

LIGHT MEALS
LIGHT MEAL 250 cal + LIGHT MEAL 250 cal + LIGHT MEAL 250 cal

OR

MAIN MEAL & SNACKS
MAIN MEAL 500 cal + SNACK 125 cal + SNACK 125 cal

NON-FAST DAYS: 1500 CALORIES

| MAINS, LIGHT MEALS & SNACKS | MAIN MEAL 500 cal | + | MAIN MEAL 500 cal | + | LIGHT MEAL 250 cal | + | SNACK 125 cal | + | SNACK 125 cal |

OR

| MAIN MEALS | MAIN MEAL 500 cal | + | MAIN MEAL 500 cal | + | MAIN MEAL 500 cal |

NON-FAST DAYS: 1800 CALORIES

| MAIN MEAL & SNACKS | MAIN MEAL 500 cal | + | MAIN MEAL 500 cal | + | MAIN MEAL 500 cal | + | SNACK 125 cal | + | SNACK 125 cal |

NON-FAST DAYS: 2000 CALORIES

| MAIN MEAL & SNACKS | MAIN MEAL 500 cal | + | MAIN MEAL 500 cal | + | MAIN MEAL 500 cal | + | SNACK 125 cal | + | SNACK 125 cal |

SNACK 125 cal + SNACK 125 cal

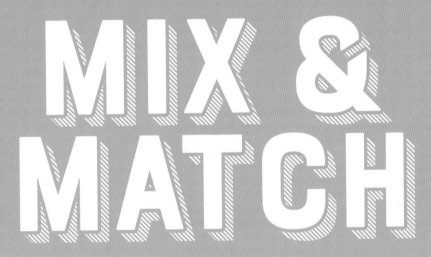

MIX & MATCH

THIS AT-A-GLANCE GUIDE WILL MAKE IT EASY
TO PLAN A SATISFYING MENU EACH DAY.

MAIN MEALS

At 500 calories or less, these will form the core of your Fast Revolution eating plan.

VG VEGETARIAN   **V** VEGAN   **GF** GLUTEN FREE   **MA** MAKE AHEAD   **F** FREEZABLE

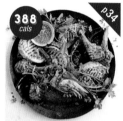
388 cals — p34
LAMB CUTLETS & SALSA VERDE
GF

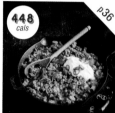
448 cals — p36
HEALTHY CHILLI CON CARNE
GF **MA** **F**

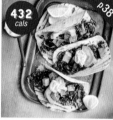
432 cals — p38
VEGAN PUMPKIN TACOS
VG **V** **GF**

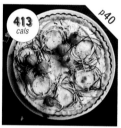
413 cals — p40
ZUCCHINI & POLENTA TART
VG **GF**

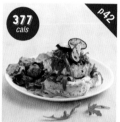
377 cals — p42
CHICKEN BURGER
MA

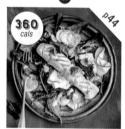
360 cals — p44
BARBECUED SALMON
GF

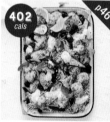
402 cals — p46
TURMERIC VEG & BUCKWHEAT
VG **GF**

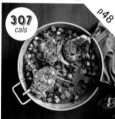
307 cals — p48
PORK & BLACK BEAN ONE-POT
GF **MA** **F**

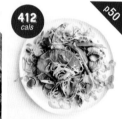
412 cals — p50
MISO PUMPKIN & BEEF NOODLES

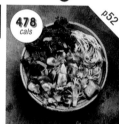
478 cals — p52
SALMON, KALE & MUSHROOM

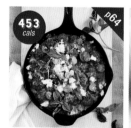
326 cals — p54
CHARGRILLED LAMB SANDWICH

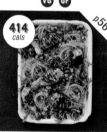
414 cals — p56
BBQ DRUMSTICKS & CARROTS
GF

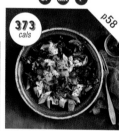
373 cals — p58
LENTIL PENNE WITH PUMPKIN
VG **V** **GF**

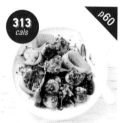
313 cals — p60
SPICY PORK MEATBALLS & QUINOA
GF **MA**

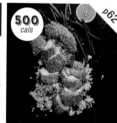
500 cals — p62
SCHNITZEL & CAULIFLOWER RICE
GF **MA** **F**

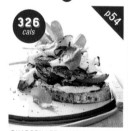
453 cals — p64
CHEESY BEEF & LENTIL MEATBALLS
GF **MA** **F**

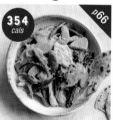
354 cals — p66
LIGHT CHICKEN KORMA
MA **F**

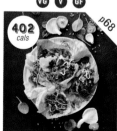
402 cals — p68
PORK SAN CHOY BAU SALAD

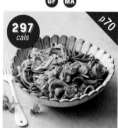
297 cals — p70
HEALTHIER BEEF STROGANOFF
GF

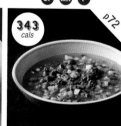
343 cals — p72
QUINOA MINESTRONE
GF **MA** **F**

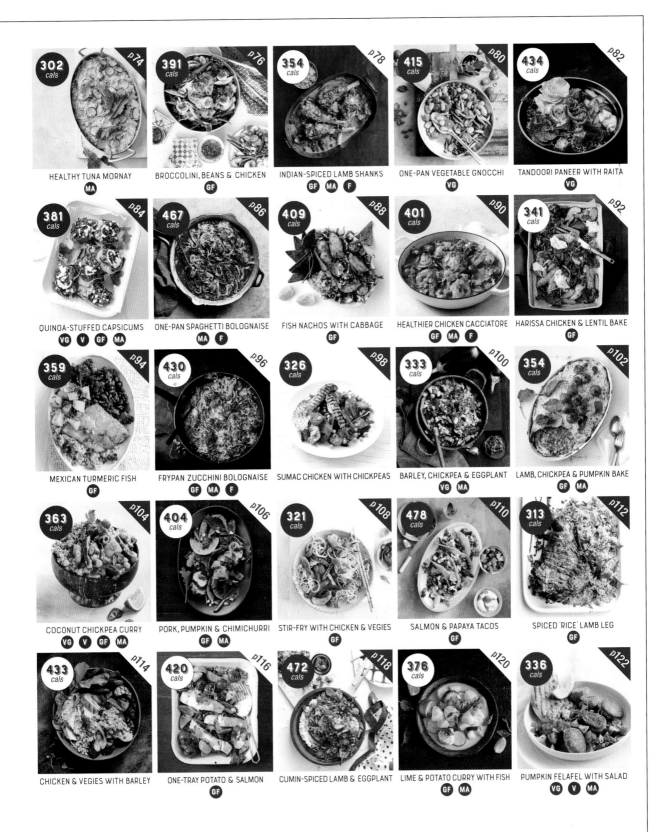

302 cals — p74
HEALTHY TUNA MORNAY
MA

391 cals — p76
BROCCOLINI, BEANS & CHICKEN
GF

354 cals — p78
INDIAN-SPICED LAMB SHANKS
GF MA F

415 cals — p80
ONE-PAN VEGETABLE GNOCCHI
VG

434 cals — p82
TANDOORI PANEER WITH RAITA
VG

381 cals — p84
QUINOA-STUFFED CAPSICUMS
VG V GF MA

467 cals — p86
ONE-PAN SPAGHETTI BOLOGNAISE
MA F

409 cals — p88
FISH NACHOS WITH CABBAGE
GF

401 cals — p90
HEALTHIER CHICKEN CACCIATORE
GF MA F

341 cals — p92
HARISSA CHICKEN & LENTIL BAKE
GF

359 cals — p94
MEXICAN TURMERIC FISH
GF

430 cals — p96
FRYPAN ZUCCHINI BOLOGNAISE
GF MA F

326 cals — p98
SUMAC CHICKEN WITH CHICKPEAS

333 cals — p100
BARLEY, CHICKPEA & EGGPLANT
VG MA

354 cals — p102
LAMB, CHICKPEA & PUMPKIN BAKE
GF MA

363 cals — p104
COCONUT CHICKPEA CURRY
VG V GF MA

404 cals — p106
PORK, PUMPKIN & CHIMICHURRI
GF MA

321 cals — p108
STIR-FRY WITH CHICKEN & VEGIES
GF

478 cals — p110
SALMON & PAPAYA TACOS
GF

313 cals — p112
SPICED 'RICE' LAMB LEG
GF

433 cals — p114
CHICKEN & VEGIES WITH BARLEY

420 cals — p116
ONE-TRAY POTATO & SALMON
GF

472 cals — p118
CUMIN-SPICED LAMB & EGGPLANT

376 cals — p120
LIME & POTATO CURRY WITH FISH
GF MA

336 cals — p122
PUMPKIN FELAFEL WITH SALAD
VG V MA

LIGHT MEALS

At around 250 calories per serve, these are great options for fasting days.

VG VEGETARIAN   **V** VEGAN   **GF** GLUTEN FREE   **MA** MAKE AHEAD   **F** FREEZABLE

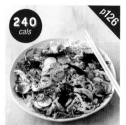

240 cals — p126

JAPANESE-STYLE CHICKEN SALAD

233 cals — p128

SALAD WITH EGG & RELISH
VG **GF**

261 cals — p130

SPICY KOREAN PORK
GF

276 cals — p132

CHICKEN & ZUCCHINI 'LINGUINE'
GF

225 cals — p134

VEGIE & GOAT'S CHEESE FRITTATA
VG **GF**

256 cals — p136

KALE WITH EGG & SWEET POTATO
VG **GF**

298 cals — p138

WHITE BEAN PANCAKES & BERRIES
VG

196 cals — p140

BARLEY, GINGER & MISO SOUP
V

192 cals — p142

ZUCCHINI SUPERFOOD SLICE
GF **MA**

270 cals — p144

ROSEMARY & LEMON STEAK
GF

197 cals — p146

SOUP WITH LEMON & TURMERIC
VG **V** **GF** **MA** **F**

253 cals — p148

SAVOURY FRENCH TOAST
VG

188 cals — p150

WATERMELON & BERRY SALAD
VG **GF**

267 cals — p152

STICKY PORK WITH ZOODLES

238 cals — p154

EGGPLANT WITH PISTACHIO & MINT
VG **V** **GF**

253 cals — p156

SOUP WITH CHICKEN & QUINOA
GF **MA** **F**

267 cals — p158

BANANA & BLUEBERRY TOAST
VG **V**

275 cals — p160

STICKY BEEF & BEAN STIR-FRY

300 cals — p162

PIRI PIRI FISH & CHARRED CORN
GF **MA** **F**

265 cals — p164

SUMMER VEG LASAGNE
VG **GF** **MA**

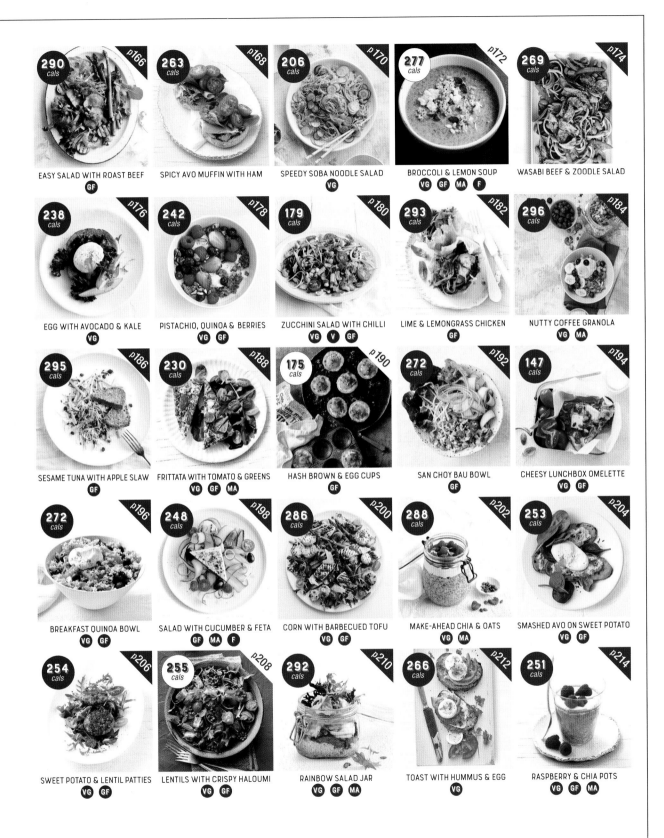

290 cals — p166
EASY SALAD WITH ROAST BEEF
GF

263 cals — p168
SPICY AVO MUFFIN WITH HAM

206 cals — p170
SPEEDY SOBA NOODLE SALAD
VG

277 cals — p172
BROCCOLI & LEMON SOUP
VG GF MA F

269 cals — p174
WASABI BEEF & ZOODLE SALAD

238 cals — p176
EGG WITH AVOCADO & KALE
VG

242 cals — p178
PISTACHIO, QUINOA & BERRIES
VG GF

179 cals — p180
ZUCCHINI SALAD WITH CHILLI
VG V GF

293 cals — p182
LIME & LEMONGRASS CHICKEN
GF

296 cals — p184
NUTTY COFFEE GRANOLA
VG MA

295 cals — p186
SESAME TUNA WITH APPLE SLAW
GF

230 cals — p188
FRITTATA WITH TOMATO & GREENS
VG GF MA

175 cals — p190
HASH BROWN & EGG CUPS
GF

272 cals — p192
SAN CHOY BAU BOWL
GF

147 cals — p194
CHEESY LUNCHBOX OMELETTE
VG GF

272 cals — p196
BREAKFAST QUINOA BOWL
VG GF

248 cals — p198
SALAD WITH CUCUMBER & FETA
GF MA F

286 cals — p200
CORN WITH BARBECUED TOFU
VG GF

288 cals — p202
MAKE-AHEAD CHIA & OATS
VG MA

253 cals — p204
SMASHED AVO ON SWEET POTATO
VG GF

254 cals — p206
SWEET POTATO & LENTIL PATTIES
VG GF

255 cals — p208
LENTILS WITH CRISPY HALOUMI
VG GF

292 cals — p210
RAINBOW SALAD JAR
VG GF MA

266 cals — p212
TOAST WITH HUMMUS & EGG
VG

251 cals — p214
RASPBERRY & CHIA POTS
VG GF MA

SNACKS

Fill the gaps in your appetite with low-cal sweets and snacks.

VG VEGETARIAN **V** VEGAN **GF** GLUTEN FREE **MA** MAKE AHEAD **F** FREEZABLE

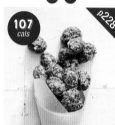
106 cals p218
MINI TUNA & CORN FRITTATAS
MA **F**

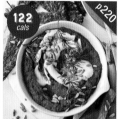
122 cals p220
ROASTED BEETROOT HUMMUS
VG **GF** **MA**

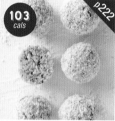
103 cals p222
SATAY BROWN RICE BALLS
VG **V** **GF** **MA**

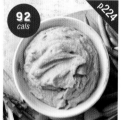
92 cals p224
BROAD BEAN & AVOCADO DIP
VG **GF** **MA**

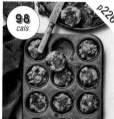
98 cals p226
VEGIE MUFFIN-PAN FRITTERS
VG

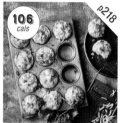
107 cals p228
BROCCOLI QUINOA NUGGETS
VG **GF**

85 cals p228
SPICED CHICKPEAS & EDAMAME
V **GF** **MA**

77 cals p229
GREEN POWER SLUSHIE
VG **GF** **MA**

82 cals p229
CREAMY LEMON & WHITE BEAN DIP
V **GF** **MA**

65 cals p230
FROZEN RASPBERRY MARBLE BITES
VG **MA** **F**

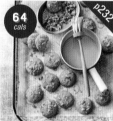
64 cals p232
HONEY & WALNUT GINGIES
VG **MA** **F**

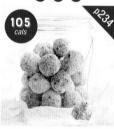
105 cals p234
TROPICAL COCONUT TREATS
VG **V** **GF** **MA**

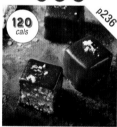
120 cals p236
CARAMEL & SESAME 'FUDGE'
VG **V** **GF** **MA**

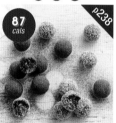
87 cals p238
MILO BLISS BALLS
VG **MA**

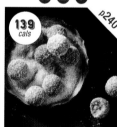
139 cals p240
PEACH & MACADAMIA BOMBS
V **GF** **MA**

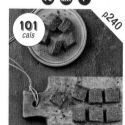
101 cals p240
DAIRY-FREE CHOC SLICE
V **GF** **MA**

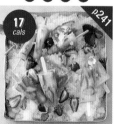
17 cals p241
EASY STRAWBERRY ICE-POPS
V **GF** **MA** **F**

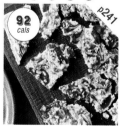
92 cals p241
BERRY GRANOLA FRO-YO BARK
VG **MA** **F**

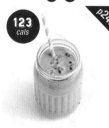
123 cals p242
TROPICAL KALE SMOOTHIE
V **GF** **MA**

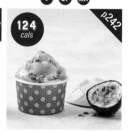
124 cals p242
PEACH & MANGO NICE CREAM
V **GF** **MA** **F**

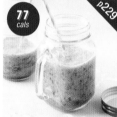
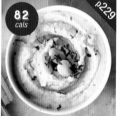
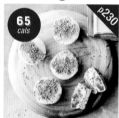
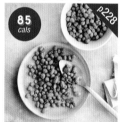

CALORIE CHART

Keep track of your calories with this handy guide that includes fruit, vegies and other easy snacks. We've even included wine and coffee.

FOOD	CALS
Fruit	
apricot	24
avocado, ½	110
banana	92
blueberries, 1 cup	73
cherries, 10	42
grapes, 1 cup	131
kiwifruit	43
mandarin	35
mango, ½	83
orange	67
pear	117
plum	25
red apple	95
strawberries, 6 large	34
watermelon, 1 cup diced	51
Vegetables	
asparagus (steamed), 8 spears	22
baby spinach, 1 cup	5
broccoli (steamed), ½ cup	26
broccolini, 4 florets	29
carrot (raw)	45
cauliflower (steamed), ½ cup	17
celery sticks (raw), 2	13
cherry tomatoes, 10	12
corncob (steamed), ½	69
green beans (steamed), ½ cup	19
new potatoes, 2	92
red cabbage (raw), 1 cup	92
red capsicum (raw), ½	38
sweet potato (steamed), 1 small	138
zucchini (steamed)	30

FOOD	CALS
Grains & Cereals	
basmati rice, ½ cup cooked	111
brown rice, ½ cup cooked	138
couscous, ½ cup cooked	128
muesli (untoasted), ⅓ cup	156
quinoa, ½ cup cooked	84
rolled oats, ⅓ cup	107
wholegrain bread roll	171
wholegrain sourdough bread, 1 slice	91
wholemeal pasta, ½ cup cooked	111

DRINKS	CALS
beer, 330ml	121
flat white coffee, 1 small takeaway	157
fresh orange juice, 1 cup	110
fresh apple juice, 1 cup	147
red wine, 150ml	115
skim flat white coffee, 1 small takeaway	84
skim milk, 1 cup	86
unsweetened almond milk, 1 cup	40
unsweetened coconut milk (carton), 1 cup	62
white wine, 150ml	111

SNACKS	CALS
almonds (roasted & unsalted), 30g	183
brown rice crackers, 10	107
carrot with 2 tbs hummus	153
carrot with 2 tbs tzatziki	74
cashews (roasted & unsalted), 30g	185
cheddar, 20g, with 6 rice crackers	144
chickpeas (roasted), 25g pkt	100
dark chocolate (70% cocoa), 25g	144
egg (boiled)	64
macadamias (roasted & unsalted), 30g	220
multigrain corn thins, 2, with 2 tsp peanut butter	122
multigrain corn thins, 2, with ¼ avocado	102
natural yoghurt, 150g, with 4 strawberries	129
potato crisps, 1 small pkt	104
popcorn with sea salt, 1 small bag	88
pretzels (salted), 1 small pkt	108
protein balls, 3	155
vanilla ice-cream, 1 medium scoop	124
wholegrain bread, 1 slice, with 2 tsp peanut butter	166
wholemeal sandwich thin, ½, with 1 tbs ricotta & 1 tomato sliced	104

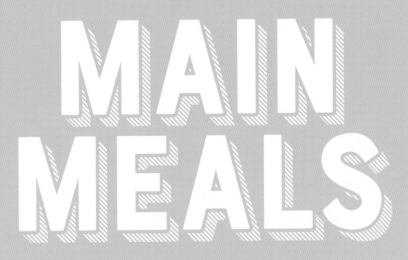

MAIN MEALS

ALL UNDER 500 CALORIES, THESE CLEVER
DISHES WILL KEEP YOU FULLER FOR LONGER.

LAMB CUTLETS WITH SALSA VERDE

Create these gluten-free lamb cutlets in just 17 minutes. The chargrilled cabbage wedges make for a budget-friendly and easy side.

SERVES 4 **PREP** 7 mins **COOK** 10 mins

8 (about 600g) large lamb cutlets
½ small savoy cabbage, cut into wedges, core intact
½ small red cabbage, cut into wedges, core intact
Rocket, to serve

SALSA VERDE
140g Sicilian olives, pitted, finely chopped
1 lemon, rind finely grated, juiced
2 tbs olive oil
1 tbs chopped fresh continental parsley or lemon thyme
1 tbs chopped capers
1 garlic clove, crushed

1 Preheat a barbecue grill or chargrill pan on high. Spray lightly with oil. Season the lamb cutlets and cook for 2-3 minutes each side or until cooked to your liking. Transfer to a plate and cover loosely with foil to keep warm.

2 Spray the cabbage with oil and chargrill for 1-2 minutes each side or until just tender.

3 Meanwhile, to make the salsa verde, put olives, lemon rind, 1-2 tbs lemon juice (to taste), oil, parsley or thyme, capers and garlic in a bowl. Season and stir to combine.

4 Arrange the lamb cutlets, cabbage and rocket on a serving platter. Spoon over the salsa verde.

NON-FAST DAYS

Add 500g baby potatoes, boiled until tender, in step 4. 81 cals per serve.

NUTRITION (PER SERVE)

CALS	FAT	SAT FAT	PROTEIN	CARBS
388	29g	9g	23g	5g

★★★★★ *Really lovely flavours.* **FRIDGETUNER**

○ VEGETARIAN · ○ VEGAN · ● GLUTEN FREE · ○ MAKE AHEAD · ○ FREEZABLE

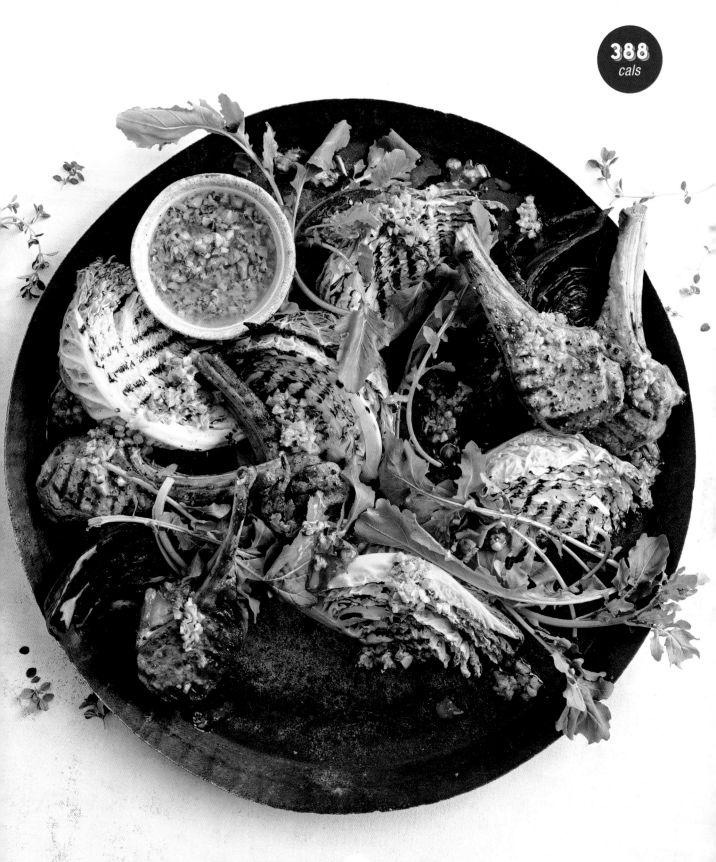

388 cals

HEALTHY CHILLI CON CARNE

Ready in 40 minutes, this healthy Mexican beef chilli is packed with vegies and served with natural yoghurt.

SERVES 4   **PREP** 10 mins   **COOK** 30 mins

1 tbs olive oil
1 brown onion, finely chopped
2 celery sticks, finely chopped
500g extra lean beef mince
3 tsp Mexican spice mix
2 tsp ground cumin
115g (½ cup) red lentils
400g can diced tomatoes
120g chargrilled capsicum
   strips, drained
400g can black beans or kidney
   beans, rinsed, drained
½ cup chopped fresh coriander
2 fresh long green chillies, sliced
Natural yoghurt, to serve (optional)

1 Heat the oil in a large heavy-based pan over medium-high heat. Add onion and celery, and cook, stirring, for 1-2 minutes. Add mince and cook, breaking up any large pieces with a wooden spoon, for 4 minutes. Add the spice mix and cumin. Season well.

2 Stir in lentils and tomato. Add 375ml (1½ cups) water. Bring mixture to the boil. Reduce heat and simmer, uncovered, for 20 minutes or until the lentils are cooked and mixture has thickened.

3 Stir through the capsicum and beans, and cook for 1-2 minutes. Stir through half the coriander and half the chilli. Divide chilli con carne among bowls. Scatter with remaining coriander and chilli. Serve with yoghurt, if using.

NUTRITION (PER SERVE)

CALS	FAT	SAT FAT	PROTEIN	CARBS
448	13.5g	3.2g	43.5g	31g

★★★★★ *A family hit. Served with guacamole, it's also good wrapped as a burrito.* **CAMTER**

○ VEGETARIAN   ○ VEGAN   ● GLUTEN FREE   ● MAKE AHEAD   ● FREEZABLE

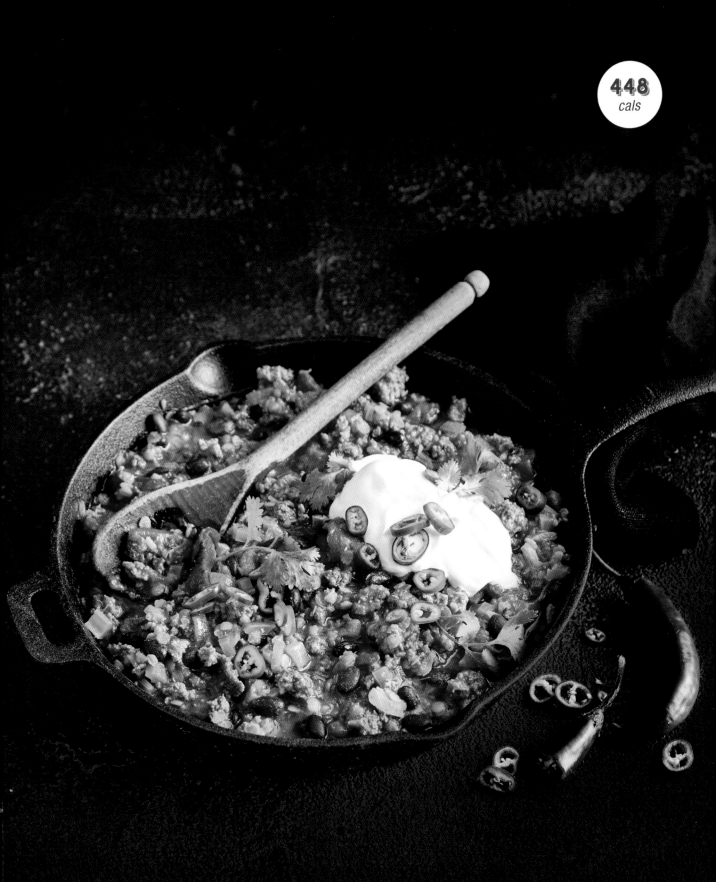

VEGAN PUMPKIN
TACOS

Using fibre-rich black beans, pumpkin and coconut yoghurt, this reinvented Mexican classic is suitable for diners of all preferences and needs.

SERVES 4 **PREP** 15 mins **COOK** 40 mins

1 tsp paprika
½ tsp dried chilli flakes
1 tsp ground cumin
500g butternut pumpkin, peeled, deseeded, cut into 2cm pieces
1 large red capsicum, deseeded, cut into 2cm pieces
400g can black beans, rinsed, drained
2 tsp pure maple syrup
2 tbs fresh lemon juice
¼ small red cabbage, shredded
95g (⅓ cup) natural coconut yoghurt
3 tsp tahini
8 small gluten-free corn tortillas
1 avocado, thinly sliced
Lemon wedges, to serve

1 Preheat oven to 200°C/180°C fan forced. Line a large baking tray with baking paper. Combine the paprika, chilli flakes and cumin in a small bowl. Place the pumpkin and capsicum on prepared tray. Lightly spray with oil. Sprinkle with the spice mixture. Roast for 30 minutes or until golden and tender, adding the black beans to the tray for the last 5 minutes of cooking. Use a fork to lightly mash the black beans after cooking.

2 Meanwhile, combine the maple syrup, 1 tbs lemon juice and a large pinch of sea salt flakes in a large bowl. Add the cabbage. Toss to combine. Set aside for 5 minutes to pickle. Drain.

3 Combine yoghurt, tahini and remaining lemon juice in a small bowl and stir until smooth. Preheat a chargrill pan over high heat. Cook tortillas for 2-3 minutes on each side.

4 Divide pickled cabbage among tortillas. Top with roast vegetables, sliced avocado and a dollop of tahini yoghurt. Season with pepper and serve with lemon wedges.

NON-FAST DAYS

Divide 120g grated vegan cheese between tacos. 81 cals per serve.

NUTRITION (PER SERVE)

CALS	FAT	SAT FAT	PROTEIN	CARBS
432	15g	4g	14g	54g

● VEGETARIAN ● VEGAN ● GLUTEN FREE ○ MAKE AHEAD ○ FREEZABLE

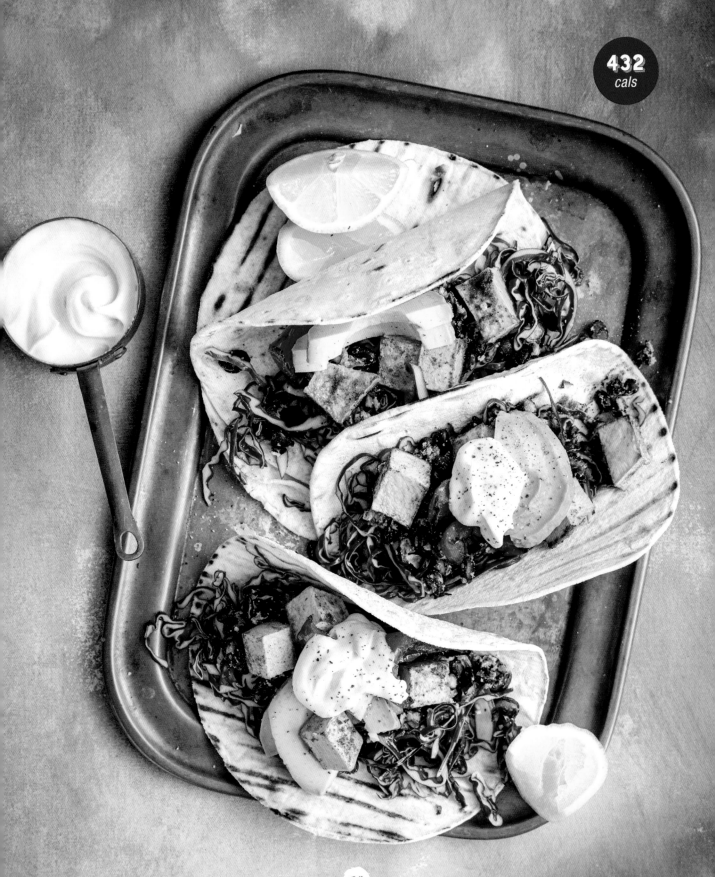

432
cals

ZUCCHINI & POLENTA TART

Serve up this healthy meat-free winner – the polenta base is a deliciously light alternative to heavy pastry.

SERVES 6   **PREP** 30 mins   **COOK** 1 hour

625ml (2½ cups) gluten-free vegetable stock
170g (1 cup) polenta
120g (1⅔ cup) shredded parmesan
2 eggs
3 zucchini, trimmed
300g fresh ricotta
150g goat's cheese
6 baby bocconcini
240g cherry truss tomatoes
Baby parsley leaves, to serve

1 Preheat the oven to 180°C/160°C fan forced. Grease a 3cm-deep, 24cm fluted tart tin with removable base.

2 Bring the stock just to a simmer in a saucepan over medium heat. Gradually add the polenta in a thin, steady stream, stirring constantly until combined. Reduce heat to medium-low and cook, stirring, for 10-15 minutes or until thickened. Remove from heat. Stir in ¾ cup of the parmesan and 1 of the eggs until well combined. Season. Press into the prepared tart tin to line the base and side. Bake for 20 minutes or until light golden and set.

3 Meanwhile, cut each zucchini in half crossways. Working with 1 piece at a time, use a spiraliser to cut the zucchini into noodles. (Alternatively, peel into ribbons, then use a knife to cut into strips). Twirl 1 portion around your fingers to make an 8cm nest. Place on a chopping board. Repeat with remaining zucchini to make 6 nests.

4 Combine the ricotta, goat's cheese, ¾ cup of the remaining parmesan and the remaining egg in a bowl. Season well. Spread into case. Top with zucchini nests. Place a bocconcini in the centre of each nest and sprinkle with the remaining parmesan.

5 Place the tart on a baking tray. Arrange tomatoes on the tray around the tart. Bake for 20-25 minutes or until cheese melts and tomatoes are just starting to collapse. Top tart with tomatoes. Sprinkle with parsley.

NUTRITION (PER SERVE)

CALS	FAT	SAT FAT	PROTEIN	CARBS
413	22g	13g	27g	24g

● VEGETARIAN   ○ VEGAN   ● GLUTEN FREE   ○ MAKE AHEAD   ○ FREEZABLE

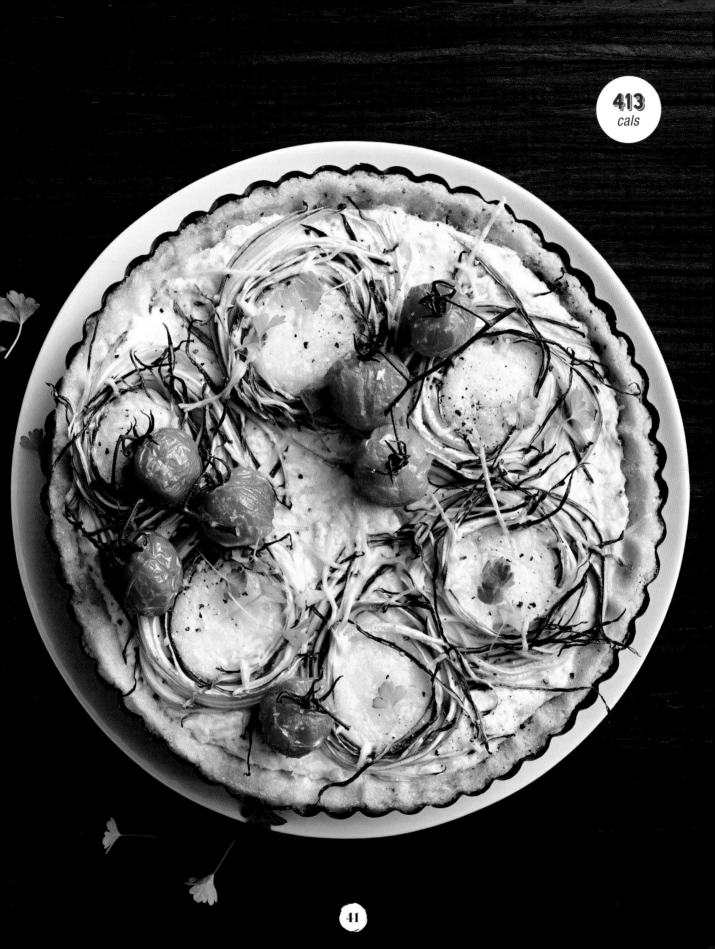

413
cals

CHICKEN BURGER

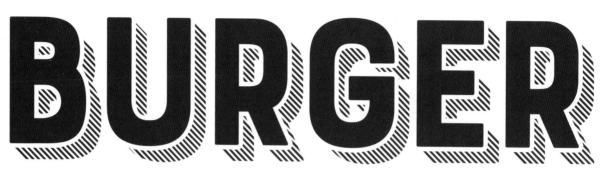

Comfort food is reinvented with this satisfying but healthier burger, accompanied by sweet potato and beetroot chips.

SERVES 4 **PREP** 20 mins **COOK** 30 mins

250g sweet potato, peeled
2 (about 250g) beetroot, peeled
1 tsp sumac
1 tsp ground cumin
3 zucchini
400g chicken breast mince
1 carrot, peeled, finely grated
3 green shallots, thinly sliced
2 tbs chopped fresh
  continental parsley
2 wholegrain bread rolls,
  halved, toasted
60g (¼ cup) bought tzatziki
Baby rocket and red sauerkraut,
  to serve

1 Preheat oven to 180°C/160°C fan forced. Line 2 baking trays with baking paper. Use a sharp knife or mandoline to thinly slice sweet potato and beetroot. Spread evenly on prepared trays. Lightly spray with oil. Sprinkle with half the sumac and half the cumin. Bake, swapping trays halfway through, for 25-30 minutes or until golden and crisp.

2 Meanwhile, finely grate 1 zucchini. Squeeze out excess moisture. Place in a bowl with chicken, carrot, shallot, parsley, remaining sumac and cumin. Season with pepper. Mix well, then shape into 4 patties.

3 Preheat a barbecue grill or large chargrill pan on medium-high. Cut each remaining zucchini lengthways into 4 slices. Lightly spray patties and zucchini with oil. Cook patties for 4-5 minutes each side or until cooked through. Cook zucchini for 1-2 minutes each side or until just tender.

4 Spread bread halves with tzatziki. Top each with rocket, a patty, sauerkraut and zucchini. Serve with sweet potato and beetroot chips.

NUTRITION (PER SERVE)

CALS	FAT	SAT FAT	PROTEIN	CARBS
377	13.5g	3.5g	27g	33g

○ VEGETARIAN ○ VEGAN ○ GLUTEN FREE ● MAKE AHEAD ○ FREEZABLE

★★★★★ These were delish. The smokiness and char from the bbq really added to the flavour. Didn't miss the deep-fried chippies and beef patties with cheese. Was a healthy Friday night! **AMCD**

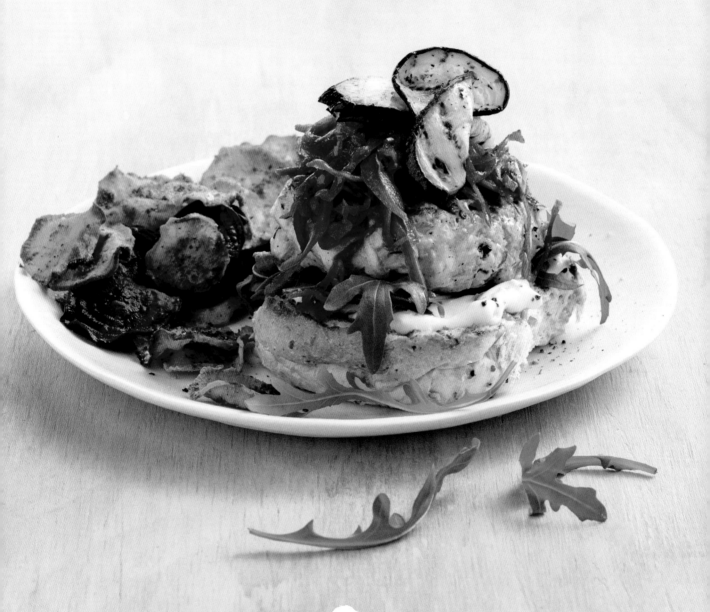

BARBECUED SALMON

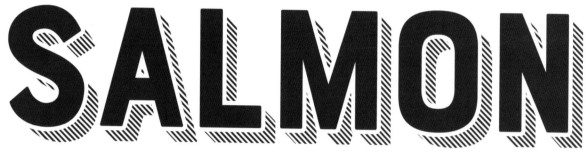

With three different types of greens and a healthy almond dressing, this salad is perfect for lazy summer evenings – and it's on the table in 20 minutes!

SERVES 4 **PREP** 10 mins **COOK** 10 mins

4 (120g each) skinless salmon fillets
2 bunches broccolini, trimmed, halved
1 tsp extra virgin olive oil
1½ tbs fresh lemon juice
2 large zucchini, peeled into ribbons
100g baby kale or mixed baby salad leaves
4 radishes, thinly sliced
1 tbs almond spread
2 tsp rice wine vinegar
2 tsp pure maple syrup
1 tsp finely grated fresh ginger
Red-vein sorrel leaves, to serve (optional)

1 Preheat a barbecue grill or chargrill pan on high. Lightly spray the salmon and broccolini with olive oil. Cook the salmon for 2-3 minutes each side or until cooked to your liking. Cook the broccolini for 2 minutes each side or until bright green and just tender.

2 Meanwhile, combine the olive oil and 2 tsp lemon juice in a large bowl. Add the zucchini ribbons and toss to coat. Season well. Add the kale and radish. Gently toss to combine.

3 Place the almond spread, rice wine vinegar, maple syrup, ginger and remaining lemon juice in a small bowl. Mix until well combined and smooth.

4 Divide the zucchini salad and grilled broccolini among serving plates. Top with the salmon and drizzle with the almond dressing. Scatter sorrel leaves over to serve, if using.

NON-FAST DAYS

Heat a 250g pkt microwave brown rice as a side. 107 cals per serve.

NUTRITION (PER SERVE)

CALS	FAT	SAT FAT	PROTEIN	CARBS
360	21g	3.5g	31.5g	8g

○ VEGETARIAN   ○ VEGAN   ● GLUTEN FREE   ○ MAKE AHEAD   ○ FREEZABLE

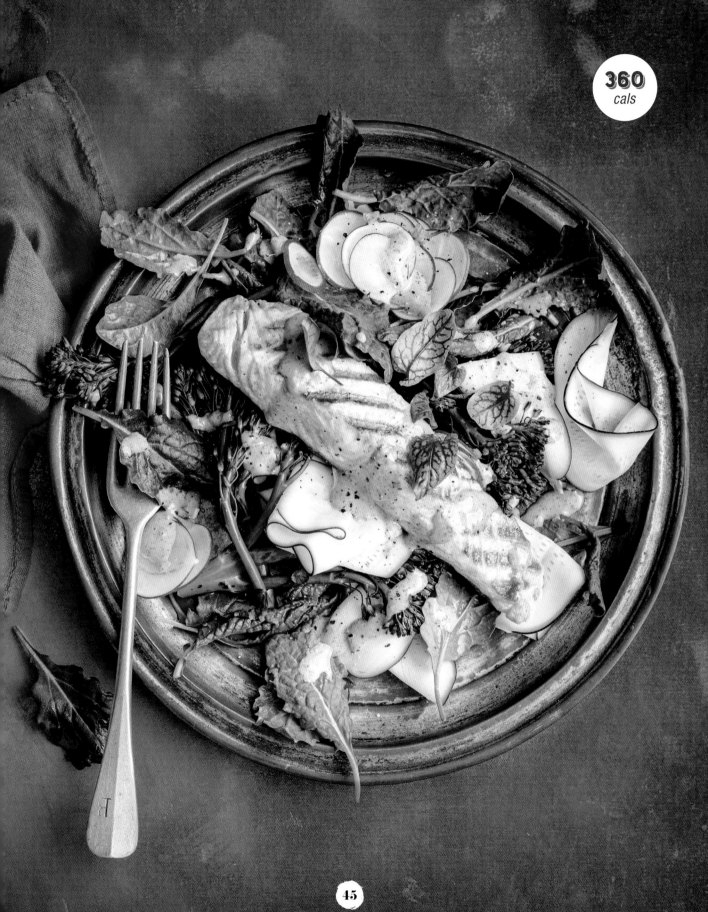

360
cals

ROAST TURMERIC VEGIES &

BUCKWHEAT

This super-simple tray bake is bursting with Middle Eastern flavours – perfect for midweek meals or weekend entertaining.

SERVES 4 **PREP** 10 mins **COOK** 25 mins

600g cauliflower, cut into florets
2 zucchini, coarsely chopped
6 Medjool dates, pitted, quartered
1 tbs olive oil
1 tbs finely grated fresh ginger
2 tsp finely grated fresh turmeric
2 garlic cloves, crushed
2 tsp ground cumin
205g (1 cup) raw buckwheat
¼ cup fresh mint sprigs
Lemon wedges, to serve
130g (½ cup) natural yoghurt

1 Preheat the oven to 200°C/180°C fan forced. Line a baking dish with baking paper. Scatter the cauliflower, zucchini and dates in prepared dish. Drizzle with the oil. Add the ginger, turmeric, garlic and cumin. Toss well to coat. Season. Roast for 25 minutes or until golden and tender.

2 Meanwhile, cook the buckwheat in a saucepan of boiling water following the packet directions. Drain.

3 Serve the roasted vegetables sprinkled with buckwheat, mint and lemon wedges, and topped with yoghurt.

NON-FAST DAYS

Mix through a 400g can of rinsed and drained chickpeas. 68 cals per serve.

NUTRITION (PER SERVE)

CALS	FAT	SAT FAT	PROTEIN	CARBS
402	8g	2g	14g	60g

● VEGETARIAN   ○ VEGAN   ● GLUTEN FREE   ○ MAKE AHEAD   ○ FREEZABLE

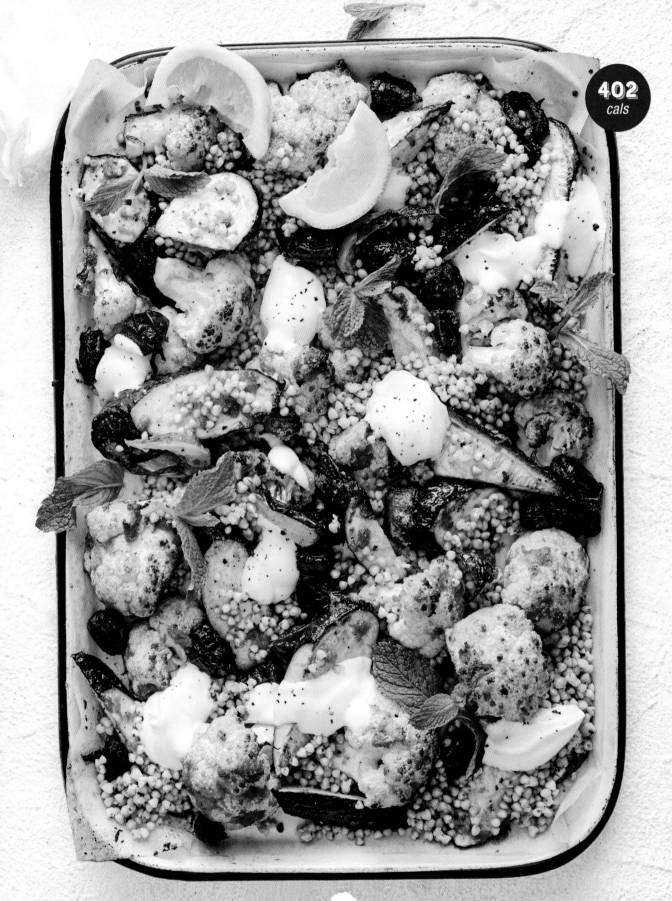

402
cals

PORK & BLACK BEAN ONE-POT

Heat up the kitchen with this one-pot favourite, which includes a delectably spicy green chilli salsa.

SERVES 4 **PREP** 10 mins **COOK** 25 mins

1½ tbs extra virgin olive oil
4 x 125g French-cut pork cutlets, fat trimmed
1 red onion, finely chopped
2 garlic cloves, crushed
1 tsp smoked paprika
1 tsp ground coriander
1 lime, rind finely grated, juiced
1 red capsicum, deseeded, finely chopped
250g sweet potato, peeled, finely chopped
1 large zucchini, chopped
400g can black beans, rinsed, drained
250ml (1 cup) gluten-free, salt-reduced chicken stock
⅓ cup fresh coriander leaves, chopped
1 fresh long green chilli, thinly sliced

1 Heat 1 tbs oil in a large non-stick frying pan over medium-high heat. Cook pork for 2-3 minutes each side or until golden. Transfer to a plate and set aside.

2 Reduce heat to medium. Add the onion to pan. Cook, stirring, for 3-4 minutes or until softened. Add the garlic, paprika, ground coriander and 1 tsp lime rind. Cook, stirring, for 1 minute or until softened. Add the capsicum, sweet potato and zucchini. Cook, stirring, for 1 minute.

3 Add black beans and stock. Bring to boil. Reduce heat. Simmer, partially covered, for 6-7 minutes. Add pork and simmer, uncovered, for 5 minutes or until vegetables are tender and pork is just cooked.

4 Meanwhile, combine the coriander leaves, lime juice, chilli, and remaining lime rind and oil. Season. Serve pork topped with the chilli salsa.

NON-FAST DAYS

Serve with
1 slice multigrain
gluten-free bread.
91 cals per serve.

NUTRITION (PER SERVE)

CALS	FAT	SAT FAT	PROTEIN	CARBS
307	9.5g	2g	30g	19g

○ VEGETARIAN ○ VEGAN ● GLUTEN FREE ● MAKE AHEAD ● FREEZABLE

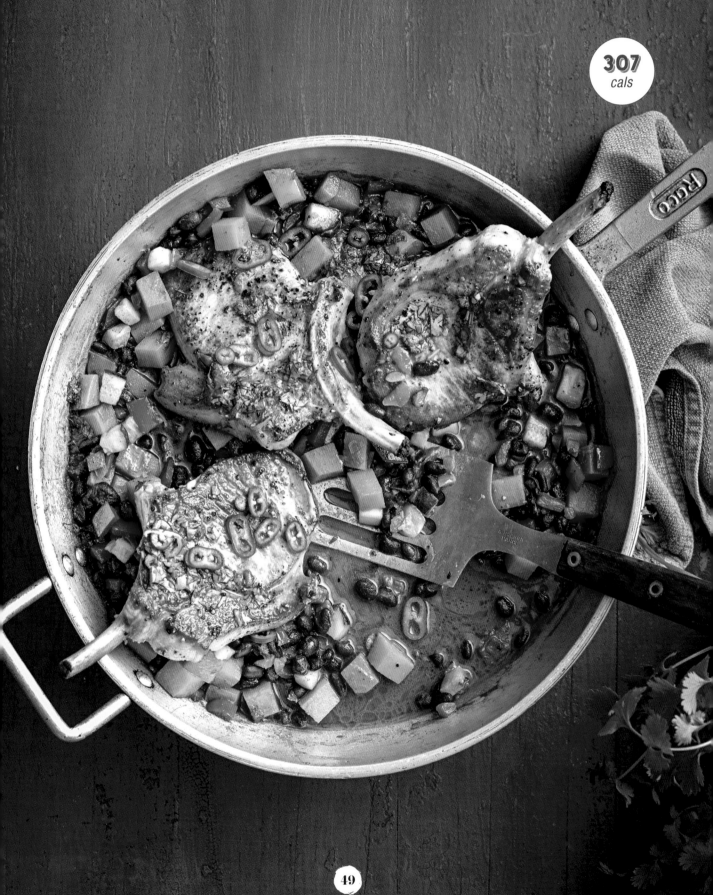

307
cals

MISO PUMPKIN & BEEF NOODLES

Low-cal and low-fat, this zingy salad looks fantastic and is super simple to pull together for a weeknight meal.

SERVES 4 **PREP** 10 mins (+ resting) **COOK** 35 mins

1kg piece kent pumpkin, deseeded,
   cut into wedges
60ml (¼ cup) mirin seasoning
2 tbs white miso paste
1 tbs rice wine vinegar
1½ tsp wasabi paste
1 tsp honey
90g dried soba noodles
350g piece beef Scotch fillet steak
200g snow peas, trimmed, cut in half
   diagonally, blanched
50g snow pea sprouts, trimmed
50g (¼ cup) pickled ginger
2 green shallots, thinly
   sliced diagonally

1 Preheat oven to 200°C/180°C fan forced. Line a baking tray with baking paper. Place pumpkin on prepared tray. Spray with olive oil. Season. Roast for 10 minutes.

2 Whisk together the mirin, miso, vinegar, wasabi and honey in a bowl. Drizzle 1½ tbs mirin mixture over the pumpkin. Roast, turning once, for 20-25 minutes, until golden and tender.

3 Meanwhile, cook noodles in a saucepan of boiling water following packet directions. Drain. Refresh under cold running water. Transfer to a bowl.

4 Heat a non-stick frying pan over medium-high heat. Spray steak with olive oil, then season. Cook, turning, for 4 minutes. Drizzle with 2 tsp dressing and cook for a further 2 minutes for medium-rare or until cooked to your liking. Set aside to rest for 4 minutes. Thinly slice.

5 Add snow peas, sprouts, ginger, shallot and beef to the noodles. Add half the remaining dressing and toss to combine. Place pumpkin on a plate. Top with the noodle mixture. Drizzle with remaining dressing.

NON-FAST DAYS

Increase beef to 500g and noodles to 180g. 147 cals per serve.

NUTRITION (PER SERVE)

CALS	FAT	SAT FAT	PROTEIN	CARBS
412	8g	3g	29g	47g

○ VEGETARIAN ○ VEGAN ○ GLUTEN FREE ○ MAKE AHEAD ○ FREEZABLE

★★★★★ *This salad is fantastic. It's fresh, with interesting flavours, and is pretty easy to whip up. Definitely adding this to my regulars list.* **RAMBLINGRUBY**

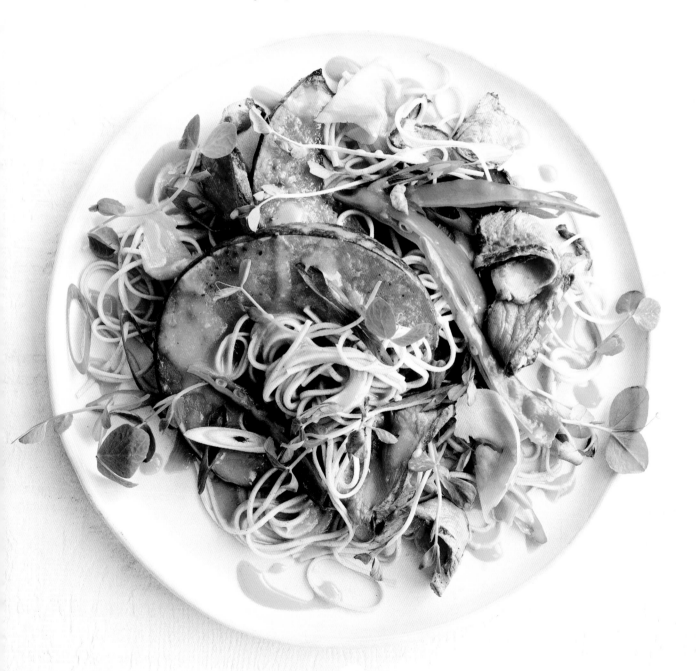

SALMON, KALE &
MUSHROOM

Japanese wasabi, soy and ginger combine with grilled salmon and delicious mushrooms to create a hearty, yet healthy lunch or dinner.

SERVES 4 **PREP** 15 mins (+ 1 hour marinating) **COOK** 15 mins

1 tsp wasabi paste
2 tbs salt-reduced soy sauce
1½ tbs mirin
1 tsp finely grated ginger
2 (175g each) skinless salmon fillets
1 tbs extra virgin olive oil
400g mixed mushrooms, quartered
1 red capsicum, deseeded, cut into thin strips
1 garlic clove, crushed
100g trimmed kale, coarsely chopped
180g dried soba noodles
Micro coriander, to serve

1 Combine the wasabi, soy sauce, mirin and ginger in a small bowl. Pour half the mixture into a shallow glass or ceramic dish, add salmon and stir to coat (reserve remaining mixture). Cover and place in the fridge for 1 hour to marinate.

2 Preheat a chargrill pan over high heat and spray lightly with oil. Grill the salmon for 2-3 minutes each side for medium or until cooked to your liking. Set aside to cool slightly, then flake the salmon.

3 Meanwhile, heat 3 tsp oil in a large non-stick frying pan over high heat. Cook mushroom, stirring, for 3 minutes or until golden. Transfer to a bowl. Set aside.

4 Heat the remaining 1 tsp oil in the frying pan. Add capsicum and garlic and cook, stirring, for 2 minutes or until just tender. Add the kale and cook, stirring, until the kale is just wilted. Remove from heat.

5 Cook the noodles in a saucepan of boiling water following the packet directions or until al dente. Drain. Divide the noodles, mushroom, capsicum mixture and salmon among bowls. Drizzle with the reserved marinade and scatter the micro coriander over to serve.

NUTRITION (PER SERVE)

CALS	FAT	SAT FAT	PROTEIN	CARBS
478	19g	4g	30g	39g

○ VEGETARIAN ○ VEGAN ○ GLUTEN FREE ○ MAKE AHEAD ○ FREEZABLE

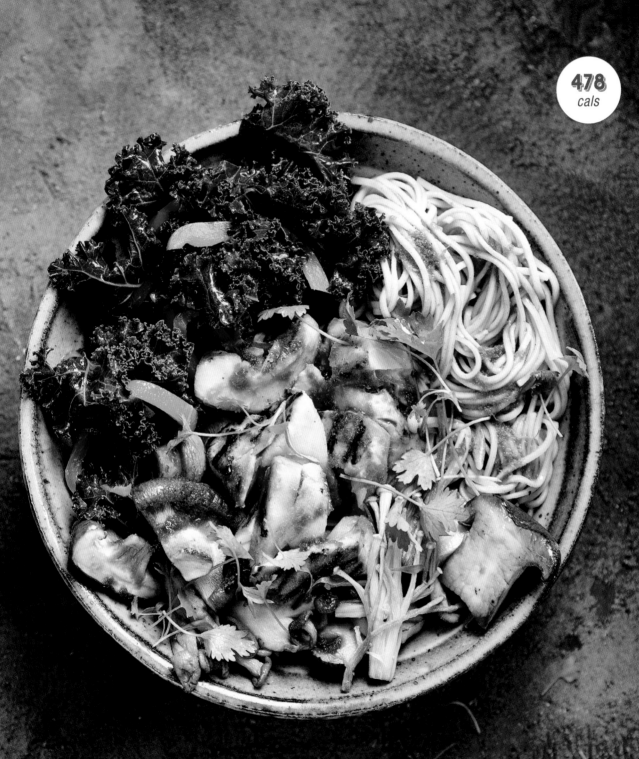

478 cals

★★★★★ *Very tasty, surprisingly filling, and exceptionally easy. This healthy, low-calorie dish is a total winner on all fronts!* **COOKINGMAMA1902**

CHARGRILLED LAMB & VEGIE
SANDWICH

Succulent lamb, spicy hummus and zucchini ribbons…
what's not to love about this mouthwatering sandwich?

SERVES 4 **PREP** 15 mins (+ 20 mins marinating) **COOK** 10 mins

400g lamb leg steaks
1 garlic clove, crushed
½ tsp ground cumin
½ tsp dried mint
1 tbs lemon juice
2 tsp extra virgin olive oil
1 large red capsicum, deseeded,
    cut into 2cm strips
1 (about 300g) eggplant, trimmed,
    cut into 1cm slices
1 large zucchini, trimmed, peeled
    into ribbons
4 slices wholegrain bread,
    chargrilled
2 tbs chilli hummus
50g baby rocket leaves, to serve
Low-fat yoghurt, to drizzle

1 Pound the lamb steaks between 2 pieces of baking paper until about 3-4mm thick. Place the garlic, cumin, mint, lemon juice and olive oil in a shallow glass or ceramic dish. Add the lamb and turn to coat. Cover and set aside for 20 minutes to marinate.

2 Preheat a chargrill pan or barbecue grill on high. Spray the capsicum, eggplant and zucchini lightly with olive oil. Chargrill the vegetables for 2-3 minutes each side or until tender and lightly charred, then transfer to a plate.

3 Chargrill the lamb for 1-2 minutes each side for medium or until cooked to your liking. Transfer to a plate. Cover with foil and set aside for 2 minutes to rest.

4 Spread bread with the hummus. Top with the eggplant, capsicum, lamb, zucchini and rocket. Drizzle with yoghurt. Season with pepper.

NON-FAST DAYS

Cut 500g sweet potato into wedges, drizzle with 1 tbs extra virgin olive oil and roast until golden to serve as a side. 128 cals per serve.

NUTRITION (PER SERVE)

CALS	FAT	SAT FAT	PROTEIN	CARBS
326	13g	3g	28g	22g

○ VEGETARIAN ○ VEGAN ○ GLUTEN FREE ○ MAKE AHEAD ○ FREEZABLE

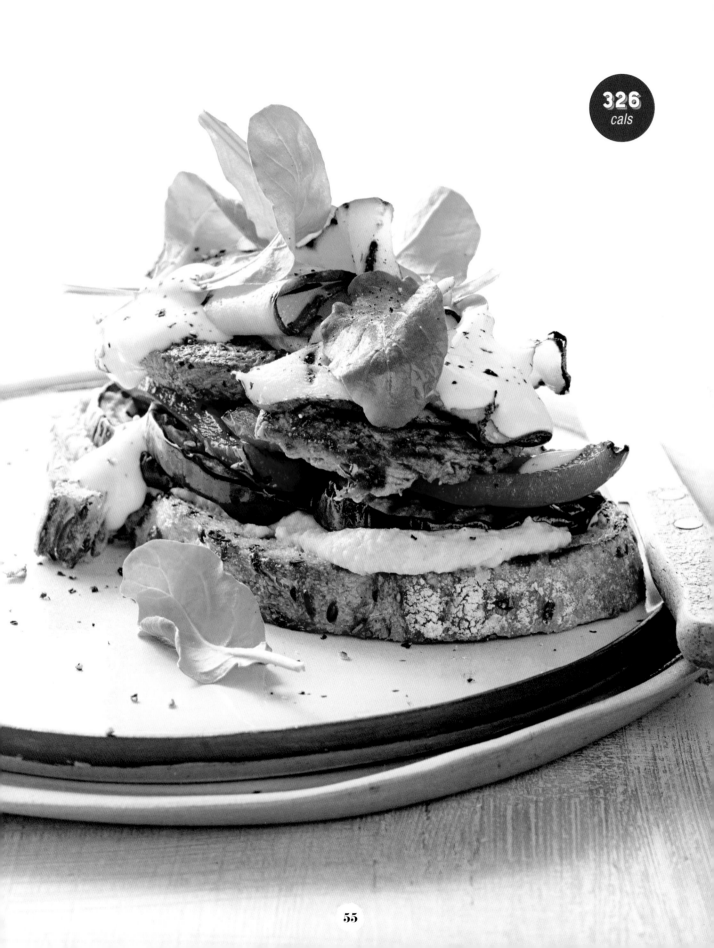

326
cals

BBQ DRUMSTICKS &

CARROTS

These deliciously sticky chargrilled chicken pieces are beautifully balanced on a colourful bed of carrots and pumpkin.

SERVES 4 **PREP** 10 mins **COOK** 45 mins

- 8 (about 1.5kg) chicken drumsticks, skin removed
- 1 tbs peri-peri seasoning
- 2 tbs chilli jam
- 500g peeled, deseeded pumpkin, finely chopped
- 2 tbs pepitas
- 60g baby rocket
- 2 carrots, peeled, cut into noodles using a spiraliser
- 2 tbs unsweetened dried cranberries

1 Lightly grease a barbecue grill or chargrill pan and preheat on high. Preheat the oven to 200°C/180°C fan forced. Slash chicken drumsticks 2-3 times on each side almost through to the bone. Combine in a bowl with peri-peri seasoning and chilli jam. Set aside.

2 Line a large baking tray with baking paper. Scatter the pumpkin over the prepared tray. Spray with oil. Season. Bake for 40-45 minutes or until golden and lightly crisp. Add pepitas to the tray for the last 5 minutes of cooking.

3 Meanwhile, barbecue or chargrill the chicken drumsticks, turning, for 20 minutes or until they are golden and cooked through.

4 Arrange the rocket, carrot, roast pumpkin and pepitas on a serving platter. Sprinkle with cranberries. Top with the drumsticks and serve immediately.

COOK'S NOTE

Serve with ½ cup (80g) steamed couscous per person. 128 cals per serve.

NUTRITION (PER SERVE)

CALS	FAT	SAT FAT	PROTEIN	CARBS
414	16g	4g	43g	22g

○ VEGETARIAN   ○ VEGAN   ● GLUTEN FREE   ○ MAKE AHEAD   ○ FREEZABLE

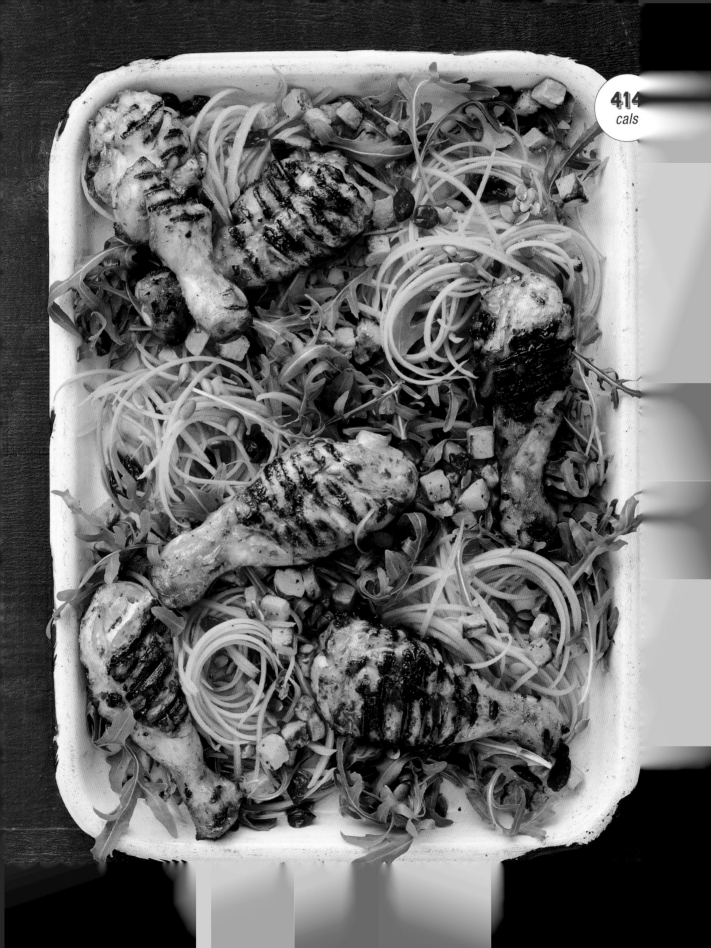

414
cals

LENTIL PENNE WITH PUMPKIN

The chilli pumpkin and tahini dressing in this recipe add spice and tang, while the kale provides green leafy goodness.

SERVES 6 **PREP** 20 mins **COOK** 35 mins

½ (about 900g) butternut pumpkin, peeled, deseeded, cut into 1.5cm pieces
1 tbs extra virgin olive oil
½ tsp cumin seeds, crushed
¼ tsp dried chilli flakes
2 cups kale leaves
250g pkt red lentil penne
Black sesame seeds, to sprinkle (optional)

TAHINI DRESSING
80ml (⅓ cup) tahini
2 tbs extra virgin olive oil
2 tbs fresh lemon juice
3 tsp apple cider vinegar
1 garlic clove, crushed
60ml (¼ cup) warm water
¼ cup finely chopped fresh coriander leaves

1 Preheat oven to 200°C/180°C fan forced. Grease 2 baking trays and line with baking paper. Place the pumpkin on 1 tray. Season with salt. Drizzle with olive oil. Bake, turning occasionally, for 25 minutes or until starting to turn golden. Sprinkle with cumin and chilli.

2 Place kale on the other prepared tray and spray with oil. Return pumpkin to oven along with kale. Bake for 10 minutes or until pumpkin is golden and kale is crisp.

3 Meanwhile, to make the tahini dressing, combine tahini, oil, lemon juice, vinegar and garlic in a small jug (mixture will seize). Stir in water until mixture loosens again. Add coriander, season and stir to combine.

4 Cook pasta in a large saucepan of boiling water following packet directions or until al dente. Add 1 tbs cooking liquid to dressing. Stir to combine. Drain pasta. Transfer to a bowl. Toss through three-quarters of the dressing. Serve pasta topped with pumpkin, kale, remaining dressing and sesame seeds, if using.

NON-FAST DAYS

Add 300g firm tofu, cut into cubes, to pumpkin in step 1. 60 cals per serve.

NUTRITION (PER SERVE)

CALS	FAT	SAT FAT	PROTEIN	CARBS
373	23.5g	2.5g	11g	35g

● VEGETARIAN ● VEGAN ● GLUTEN FREE ○ MAKE AHEAD ○ FREEZABLE

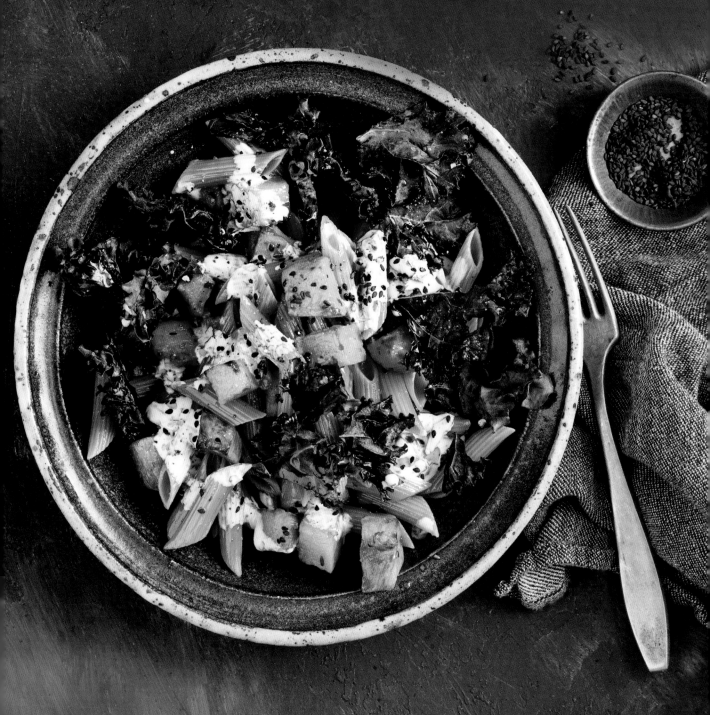

SPICY PORK MEATBALLS &
QUINOA

Fresh Asian flavours lift this dish into total deliciousness
and the lean mince makes it super-healthy too.

SERVES 4 **PREP** 15 mins **COOK** 15 mins

500g extra-lean pork mince
2 tsp finely grated fresh ginger
3 tsp sambal oelek
2 tsp fish sauce
2 tbs chopped fresh coriander,
    plus ½ cup whole leaves, extra
2 tsp extra virgin olive oil
100g baby spinach leaves
2 carrots, peeled into ribbons
1 Lebanese cucumber, peeled
    into ribbons
4 radishes, thinly sliced
1 tbs fresh lime juice
1 tsp brown sugar
3 cups (450g) cooked quinoa,
    to serve

1 Combine pork, ginger, 2 tsp sambal oelek, 1 tsp fish sauce and chopped coriander in a bowl. Roll tablespoonfuls of mixture into 24 balls. Place on a lined plate.

2 Heat 1 tsp oil in a non-stick frying pan over medium heat. Cook meatballs, in batches, turning, for 5-6 minutes, until cooked through.

3 Meanwhile, combine the spinach, carrot, cucumber, radish and extra coriander in a large bowl. Place the lime juice, sugar and remaining sambal oelek, fish sauce and oil in a small bowl. Stir until the sugar dissolves.

4 Place quinoa, spinach salad and meatballs on serving plates. Drizzle with the dressing.

NON-FAST DAYS

Boost this meal by increasing the quinoa to 4 cups. 50 cals per serve.

NUTRITION (PER SERVE)

CALS	FAT	SAT FAT	PROTEIN	CARBS
313	7g	2g	31g	27g

★★★★★ *Super easy meatballs that I prepped to take to work for lunch. My 10 year old loved the extra ones left over. We've even used the pork mixture as a filling for delicious dumplings.* **CURLY_SHIRLEY**

○ VEGETARIAN ○ VEGAN ● GLUTEN FREE ● MAKE AHEAD ○ FREEZABLE

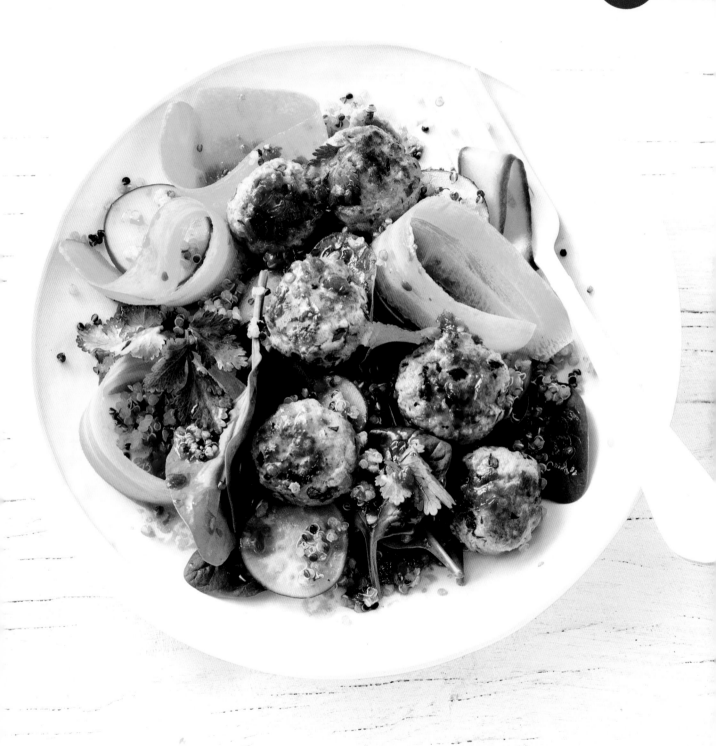

313
cals

SCHNITZEL & CAULIFLOWER RICE

The delicious seed crust on these schnitzels provides a fresh twist on a crumb, while the super-simple cauliflower rice gives the dish extra crunch.

SERVES 4 **PREP** 10 mins **COOKING** 15 mins

35g (⅓ cup) mixed seeds (chia, hemp and sesame seeds)
50g (¼ cup) polenta
20g (¼ cup) finely grated parmesan
1 egg
2 tsp arrowroot (tapioca flour)
2 large (about 300g each) chicken breasts, halved diagonally
2 tbs extra virgin olive oil
Steamed green beans, to serve

PARMESAN CAULIFLOWER RICE

1 tbs extra virgin olive oil
3 green shallots, thinly sliced, plus extra, to serve (optional)
3 garlic cloves, crushed
2 x 250g pkt cauliflower rice
1 large lemon, rind finely grated, halved
25g (⅓ cup) finely grated parmesan

1 Combine the seeds, polenta and parmesan on a plate. Season. Lightly whisk egg, 1 tbs water and arrowroot in a shallow bowl. Dip chicken pieces in egg then in the seed mixture, pressing to coat.

2 Heat the oil in a large non-stick frying pan over medium heat. Cook the chicken, turning, for 6-7 minutes or until golden and just cooked through. Transfer to a plate lined with paper towel. Wipe the pan clean with paper towel.

3 To make parmesan cauliflower rice, heat oil in pan over high heat. Add shallot and garlic. Cook, stirring, for 1 minute or until aromatic. Add cauliflower rice. Cook, stirring, for 1 minute or until coated. Add lemon rind and juice of 1 lemon half. Cook, stirring occasionally, for 2 minutes or until tender. Stir in parmesan until combined. Season.

4 Serve the cauliflower rice with the schnitzels, green beans, remaining lemon half and extra shallot, if using.

COOK'S NOTE

Chia seeds have the highest content of plant based omega-3 fatty acids.

NUTRITION (PER SERVE)

CALS	FAT	SAT FAT	PROTEIN	CARBS
500	27g	6g	46g	14.5g

○ VEGETARIAN ○ VEGAN ● GLUTEN FREE ● MAKE AHEAD ● FREEZABLE

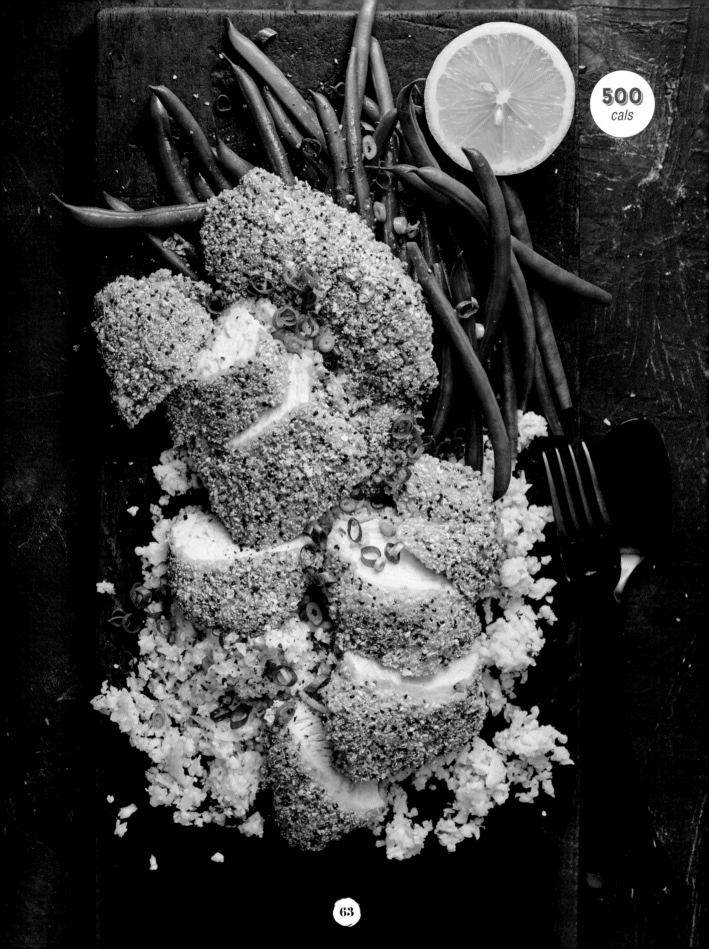

500
cals

CHEESY BEEF & LENTIL
MEATBALLS

Made with lean mince, cheese and lentils, these flavourful meatballs are both hearty and healthy.

SERVES 4 **PREP** 25 mins (+ 30 mins chilling + 5 mins standing) **COOK** 35 mins

500g lean beef mince
400g can brown lentils,
   rinsed, drained
½ red onion, finely chopped or grated
1 zucchini, coarsely grated
⅓ cup fresh basil leaves,
   finely chopped
25g (¼ cup) quinoa flakes
2 garlic cloves, crushed
1 egg, lightly whisked
2 tsp dried oregano leaves
2 tsp olive oil
500ml (2 cups) tomato passata
200g mixed baby tomatoes, halved
2 tsp balsamic vinegar
40g (⅓ cup) coarsely grated
   fresh mozzarella
75g Greek feta, crumbled
Fresh basil leaves, extra, to serve

1 Place the mince, lentils, onion, zucchini, basil, quinoa flakes, garlic, egg and 1 tsp of the oregano in a large bowl. Season well with salt and pepper. Use clean hands to mix well until combined. Roll rounded tablespoonfuls of the mixture into balls. Transfer to a lined plate. Cover with plastic wrap and place in the fridge for 30 minutes or until firm.

2 Preheat oven to 200°C/180°C fan forced. Heat the oil in a large, non-stick ovenproof frying pan over medium-high heat. Cook meatballs, turning, for 8 minutes or until browned. Remove from heat. Drizzle with tomato passata, keeping meatballs slightly exposed.

3 Combine tomato and vinegar in a bowl. Season. Spoon the tomato mixture among the meatballs. Sprinkle with mozzarella and feta. Sprinkle with remaining oregano. Bake for 25 minutes or until golden and bubbling. Stand for 5 minutes. Sprinkle with extra basil.

NUTRITION (PER SERVE)

CALS	FAT	SAT FAT	PROTEIN	CARBS
453	18g	7g	44g	23g

★★★★★ *I'm not an adventurous cook and I've a fussy husband, but we loved this dish!* **VICKIC_HAPPY**

○ VEGETARIAN   ○ VEGAN   ● GLUTEN FREE   ● MAKE AHEAD   ● FREEZABLE

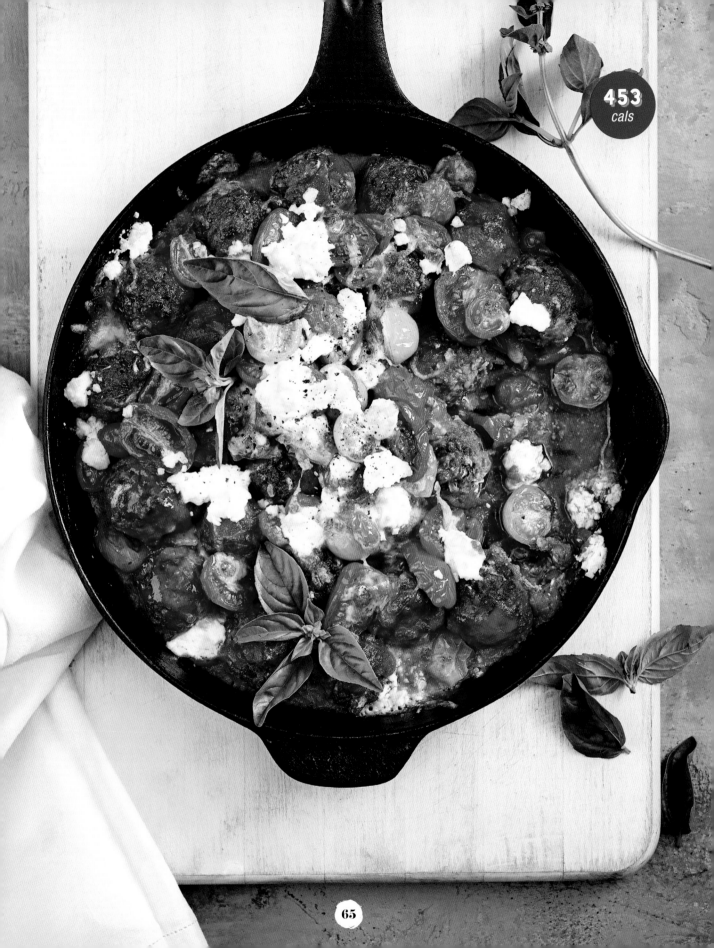

453
cals

LIGHT CHICKEN
KORMA

We have reinvented this popular curry to make it lighter in fat, but still rich in its essential flavour and spices.

SERVES 4 **PREP** 15 mins **COOK** 30 mins

2 tsp macadamia oil
500g chicken breast fillets, thinly sliced
2 brown onions, thinly sliced
2 tbs korma curry paste
1 cinnamon stick
8 cardamom pods, lightly crushed
½ tsp salt-reduced chicken stock powder
2 carrots, peeled, sliced diagonally
200g green beans, trimmed, halved
1 bunch broccolini, trimmed, cut into 4cm lengths
70g (¼ cup) natural yoghurt
1 tbs almond meal
2 (47g each) roti, warmed and halved, to serve

1 Heat 1 tsp oil in a large saucepan or wok over high heat. Cook chicken, in 2 batches, for 2-3 minutes or until browned. Transfer the chicken to a plate.

2 Heat remaining 1 tsp oil in pan or wok over high heat. Add onion and cook, stirring, for 3-4 minutes, until softened. Add the korma paste, cinnamon stick and cardamom pods. Cook, stirring, for 2 minutes or until aromatic. Add 250ml (1 cup) water. Stir in the stock powder and carrot. Return the chicken to the pan. Bring to the boil, then partially cover and reduce the heat to low. Simmer for 10 minutes or until the carrot is tender.

3 Add the beans and broccolini to the pan. Simmer for 5 minutes or until the vegetables are just tender. Remove cinnamon stick. Remove from the heat and stir through the yoghurt and almond meal. Serve with roti.

NON-FAST DAYS

Serve with
½ cup steamed
brown rice
per person.
138 cals per serve.

NUTRITION (PER SERVE)

CALS	FAT	SAT FAT	PROTEIN	CARBS
354	11g	3g	35g	22g

○ VEGETARIAN   ○ VEGAN   ○ GLUTEN FREE   ● MAKE AHEAD   ● FREEZABLE

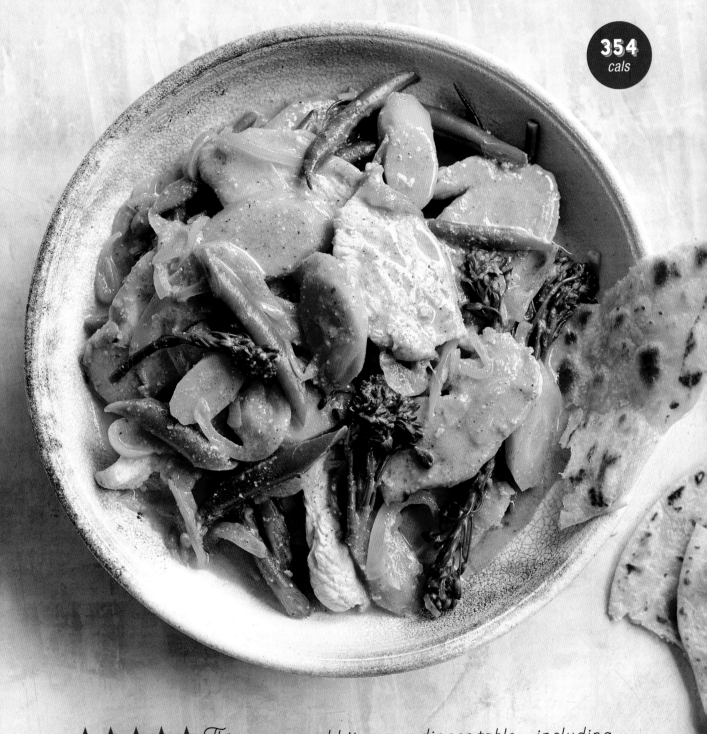

★★★★★ *This was a real hit on our dinner table – including with our children aged 6 and 9 years old. Yummy with steamed rice, naan bread and pappadams.* **FAMILY CHEF**

354 cals

PORK SAN CHOY BAU SALAD

This quick and easy twist takes all the best bits of traditional san choy bau to make a super-fresh dinner option.

SERVES 4 **PREP** 10 mins **COOK** 10 mins

2 tsp sesame oil
200g mixed mushrooms, chopped
500g lean pork and veal mince
2 garlic cloves, crushed
2 tsp finely grated fresh ginger
60ml (¼ cup) oyster sauce
100g baby spinach
250g pkt microwave 7 ancient grains
   or brown rice and chia
Butter lettuce leaves, to serve
2 green shallots, thinly sliced,
   to serve
2 tbs sunflower seeds, toasted,
   to serve
Fried shallots, to serve

1 Heat the oil in a large non-stick frying pan over medium heat. Add mushroom and cook, stirring, for 2-3 minutes or until lightly golden. Add the mince. Cook, breaking up any lumps with a wooden spoon, for 4-5 minutes or until browned.

2 Add the garlic and ginger and cook for 1 minute or until aromatic. Add the oyster sauce. Add the spinach and grains or rice. Cook, stirring, until warmed through.

3 Divide the mince mixture among lettuce leaves and arrange on a platter. Top with green shallot, sunflower seeds and fried shallots.

NON-FAST DAYS

Sprinkle ⅓ cup chopped unsalted peanuts over the mince mixture. 78 cals per serve.

NUTRITION (PER SERVE)

CALS	FAT	SAT FAT	PROTEIN	CARBS
402	14g	4g	33g	34g

★★★★★

I've made this many times on a weeknight as a quick yet tasty meal that the whole family loves. Super cheap, yet flavoursome and healthy. **ALICEH**

○ VEGETARIAN ○ VEGAN ○ GLUTEN FREE ○ MAKE AHEAD ○ FREEZABLE

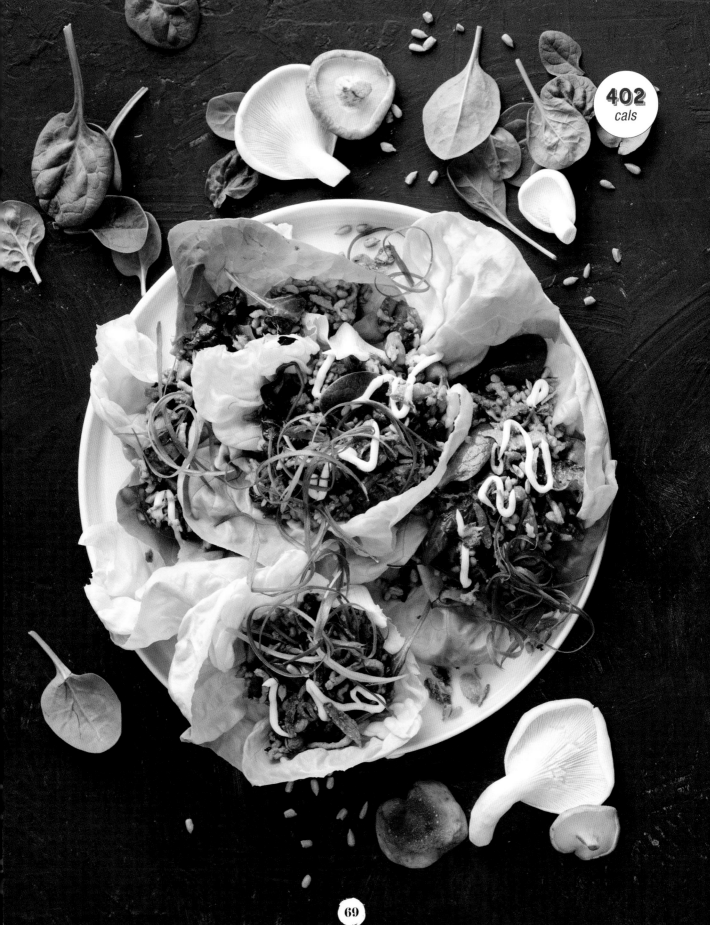

402 *cals*

HEALTHIER BEEF
STROGANOFF

We've reworked this family favourite to produce a better-for-you version. You won't notice the difference in the taste!

SERVES 4 **PREP** 20 mins **COOK** 30 mins

2 tsp olive oil
500g beef fillet, fat trimmed, thinly sliced
1 white onion, thinly sliced
200g Swiss brown mushrooms, halved or sliced
200g button mushrooms, halved or sliced
2 garlic cloves, crushed
1 tsp paprika
1 tbs gluten-free Worcestershire sauce
200ml salt-reduced gluten-free beef stock
60ml (¼ cup) reduced-fat sour cream
100g baby spinach
2 x 250g pkt zucchini noodles
Steamed green beans, to serve
Baby parsley leaves, to serve

1 Heat half the olive oil in a large non-stick frying pan over high heat. Cook the beef, in 2 batches, for 2 minutes or until golden. Transfer to a plate.

2 Heat the remaining oil in same pan over medium heat. Cook the onion, stirring, for 5 minutes or until softened. Add the mushrooms and increase heat to high. Cook, stirring, for 3-4 minutes or until browned. Add the garlic and paprika and cook, stirring, for 1 minute or until aromatic. Add the Worcestershire sauce and stock and bring to the boil.

3 Reduce heat to low, return the beef to the pan and gently simmer for 1-2 minutes or until heated through. Stir in the sour cream and spinach and cook until the spinach has just wilted.

4 Microwave the zucchini noodles following packet directions. Serve the beef with the zucchini noodles and steamed green beans, and sprinkled with the parsley.

NON-FAST DAYS

Replace the zucchini noodles with 200g dried gluten-free pasta, cooked until al dente. 156 cals per serve.

NUTRITION (PER SERVE)

CALS	FAT	SAT FAT	PROTEIN	CARBS
297	13g	5g	35g	6g

○ VEGETARIAN ○ VEGAN ● GLUTEN FREE ○ MAKE AHEAD ○ FREEZABLE

297 cals

★★★★★ *We followed this to the letter with the exception of the zucchini noodles that we made from scratch ourselves. It was so full of flavour and very healthy. Will definitely have this again, and will become one of our household regulars.* **RACHELC101**

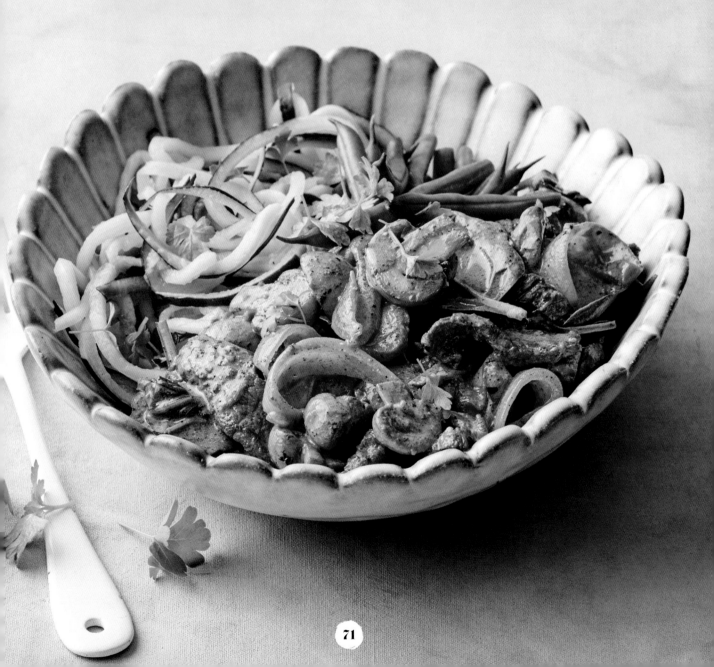

QUINOA MINESTRONE WITH KALE PESTO

Using quinoa in place of pasta adds extra protein and makes this hearty soup gluten free.

SERVES 4 **PREP** 10 mins **COOK** 25 mins

1 large brown onion,
  coarsely chopped
1 large carrot, peeled,
  coarsely chopped
1 celery stick, coarsely chopped
2 garlic cloves, halved
2 tsp extra virgin olive oil
100g pancetta, chopped
1 dried bay leaf
1L (4 cups) gluten-free chicken stock
410g can crushed tomatoes
70g (⅓ cup) tricoloured quinoa, rinsed
2 small zucchini, finely chopped
400g can borlotti beans,
  rinsed, drained

KALE PESTO
65g (2½ cups) shredded kale leaves
20g (¼ cup) finely grated parmesan
1 small garlic clove, halved
1 tbs lemon juice
1 tbs extra virgin olive oil
1 tbs water

1 Process the onion, carrot, celery and garlic in a food processor until finely chopped. Heat the oil in a saucepan over medium-low heat. Add the pancetta. Cook, stirring, for 2 minutes or until golden. Add the vegetable mixture and bay leaf. Cook, covered, stirring occasionally, for 4 minutes or until soft. Uncover and cook, stirring, for 2 more minutes.

2 Add stock and tomato to pan. Increase heat to high. Bring to the boil. Reduce heat to medium-low. Stir in quinoa. Simmer, stirring occasionally, for 5 minutes. Stir in zucchini. Cook, stirring occasionally, for 5 minutes. Add borlotti beans. Cook, stirring occasionally, for 2 minutes or until quinoa and zucchini are tender. Season with pepper.

3 For the pesto, process the kale, parmesan and garlic until finely chopped. Combine the juice, oil and water in a jug. Add juice mixture, in a slow steady stream, to kale mixture, until well combined. Season. Divide soup among bowls. Top with pesto.

NON-FAST DAYS

Serve with
1 slice multigrain
gluten-free bread.
91 cals per serve.

NUTRITION (PER SERVE)

CALS	FAT	SAT FAT	PROTEIN	CARBS
343	15g	4g	18g	32g

○ VEGETARIAN ○ VEGAN ● GLUTEN FREE ● MAKE AHEAD ● FREEZABLE

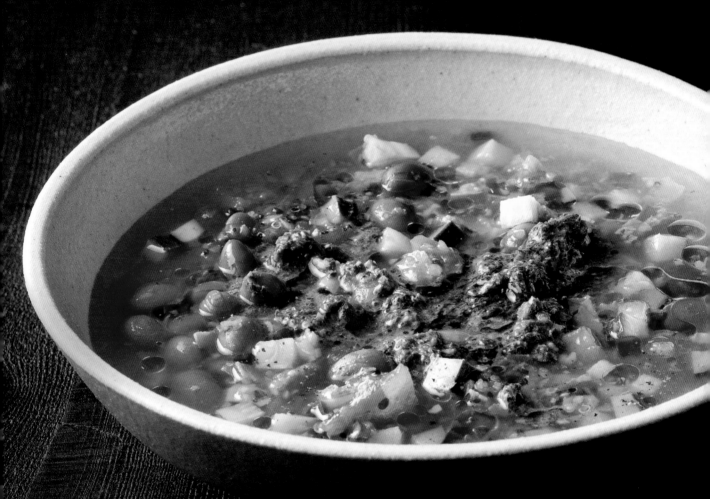

343 cals

★★★★★ This is the tastiest minestrone I've ever had, and it's so filling. The pesto is delicious too and such a great idea to use kale. Everyone loved it! SUPER_FOODIE

HEALTHY TUNA
MORNAY

We've reinvented a stodgy family classic into a newer, better-for-you bake that will soon become a light and easy favourite.

SERVES 6 **PREP** 20 mins **COOK** 30 mins

1 tsp olive oil
1 onion, finely chopped
2 celery sticks, finely chopped
1 large carrot, peeled, finely chopped
2 zucchini, thinly sliced
200g green beans, cut into
   1cm lengths
1½ tbs olive oil spread
2 tbs plain flour
500ml (2 cups) reduced-fat milk
425g can tuna in spring water,
   drained, flaked
40g (½ cup) grated parmesan
270g (2 cups) cooked brown rice
120g baby spinach leaves
Mixed salad leaves, to serve

1 Preheat oven to 190°C/170°C fan forced. Lightly spray a 2L (8-cup) ovenproof baking dish with oil.

2 Heat the oil in a large saucepan over medium heat. Cook the onion, celery and carrot, stirring, for 5 minutes or until softened. Add the zucchini and beans and cook, stirring, for 2 minutes or until just tender. Transfer the vegetables to a bowl.

3 Return same pan to medium heat and heat the spread until melted. Add the flour and stir until well combined. Slowly start adding the milk, stirring constantly, until well combined and smooth. Bring to the boil, reduce heat to low and simmer, stirring constantly, until the sauce thickens. Stir in the vegetables, tuna and half the parmesan. Season.

4 Spread the rice over base of baking dish. Top with the spinach, then the tuna mixture. Sprinkle with the remaining parmesan. Bake for 20 minutes or until golden and bubbling. Set aside for 5 minutes before serving with salad leaves.

NUTRITION (PER SERVE)

CALS	FAT	SAT FAT	PROTEIN	CARBS
302	9g	3g	22g	30g

★★★★★

This was full of easy-to-get supermarket and pantry ingredients. I'll be making it again as it was tasty, filling and healthy! **AMCD**

○ VEGETARIAN   ○ VEGAN   ○ GLUTEN FREE   ● MAKE AHEAD   ○ FREEZABLE

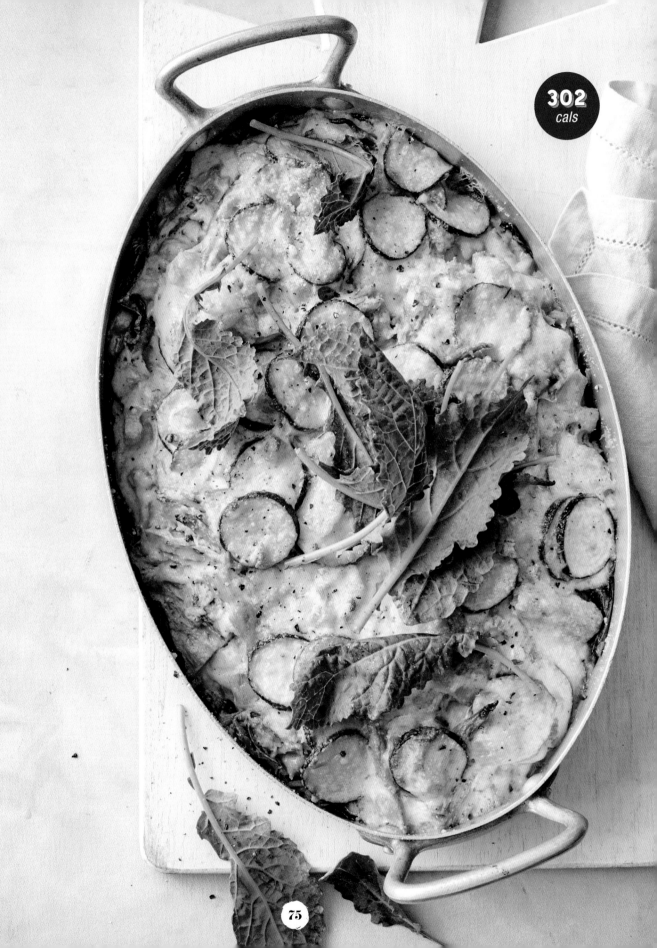

BROCCOLINI & BEAN WITH CHICKEN

This healthy and family-friendly salad uses mint and lemon to create a zesty dressing accompaniment.

SERVES 4 **PREP** 20 mins **COOK** 10 mins

1½ tbs extra virgin olive oil
1 large chicken breast fillet
150g green beans, trimmed
1 bunch broccolini, trimmed, halved lengthways
400g can cannellini beans, rinsed, drained
3 green shallots, thinly sliced
1 avocado, sliced
4 radishes, sliced
60g baby rocket
2 tbs lemon juice
1 tbs finely chopped fresh mint leaves, plus extra leaves to serve
1 tbs finely chopped pistachio kernels
4 soft-boiled eggs, halved

1 Heat 2 tsp oil in a frying pan over medium-high heat. Cook chicken for 4 minutes each side or until cooked through. Transfer to a plate. Cover loosely with foil. Stand for 5 minutes to rest. Slice.

2 Meanwhile, cook green beans and broccolini in a large saucepan of boiling water for 3 minutes or until bright green and tender. Drain. Refresh under cold water. Drain. Transfer to a large serving bowl.

3 Add cannellini beans, shallot, avocado, radish, rocket and chicken to broccolini mixture. Toss gently to combine.

4 Place lemon juice, mint, pistachios and remaining oil in a bowl. Season with salt and pepper. Stir to combine.

5 Top salad with egg and extra mint leaves. Drizzle with dressing. Serve.

NON-FAST DAYS

Serve with 1 slice gluten-free multigrain bread per person.
93 cals per serve.

NUTRITION (PER SERVE)

CALS	FAT	SAT FAT	PROTEIN	CARBS
391	22.6g	4.7g	29.8g	11.1g

○ VEGETARIAN   ○ VEGAN   ● GLUTEN FREE   ○ MAKE AHEAD   ○ FREEZABLE

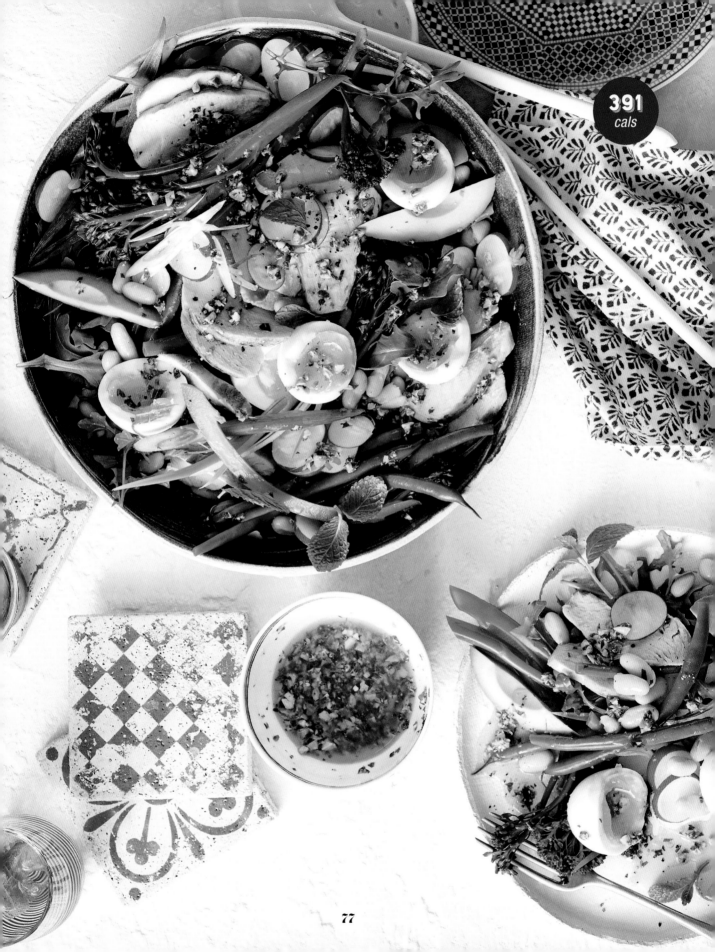

391
cals

INDIAN-SPICED LAMB
SHANKS

These flavourful Indian-inspired spiced lamb shanks are rich and satisfying. Serve with broccoli rice to soak up the sauce.

SERVES 4 **PREP** 20 mins **COOK** 2 hours 40 mins

1 tsp macadamia oil
4 small (250g each) French-trimmed
   lamb shanks
1 large red onion, finely chopped
2 celery sticks, thinly sliced
2 large carrots, peeled, thickly sliced
2 fresh long green chillies, finely
   chopped, plus extra, thinly sliced,
   to serve
3 garlic cloves, thinly sliced
2 tsp finely grated fresh ginger
2 tsp ground cumin
2 tsp ground coriander
250ml (1 cup) reduced-salt
   gluten-free chicken stock
2 tbs natural yoghurt
60g baby spinach
400g broccoli
Fresh coriander sprigs, to serve

1 Preheat oven to 160°C/140°C fan forced. Heat the oil in a large flameproof casserole dish over high heat. Add lamb. Cook, turning, for 2-3 minutes or until browned. Transfer to a plate and set aside.

2 Reduce heat to medium. Add onion, celery and carrot to casserole dish. Cook, stirring, for 5-6 minutes or until soft. Add chilli, garlic, ginger, cumin and ground coriander. Stir for 1 minute or until aromatic.

3 Return lamb to dish with stock and 250ml (1 cup) water. Bring to the boil. Roast, covered, for 2-2½ hours or until lamb is very tender. Remove lamb. Set aside. Add yoghurt and spinach to casserole dish. Stir until spinach has just wilted. Return lamb to dish.

4 Meanwhile, place the broccoli in a food processor. Process until it resembles coarse crumbs. Transfer to a microwave-safe dish. Cover and microwave on High for 2-3 minutes or until just tender. Serve lamb with coriander sprigs, extra chilli and broccoli rice.

NUTRITION (PER SERVE)

CALS	FAT	SAT FAT	PROTEIN	CARBS
354	17g	6g	37g	8g

○ VEGETARIAN ○ VEGAN ● GLUTEN FREE ● MAKE AHEAD ● FREEZABLE

354
cals

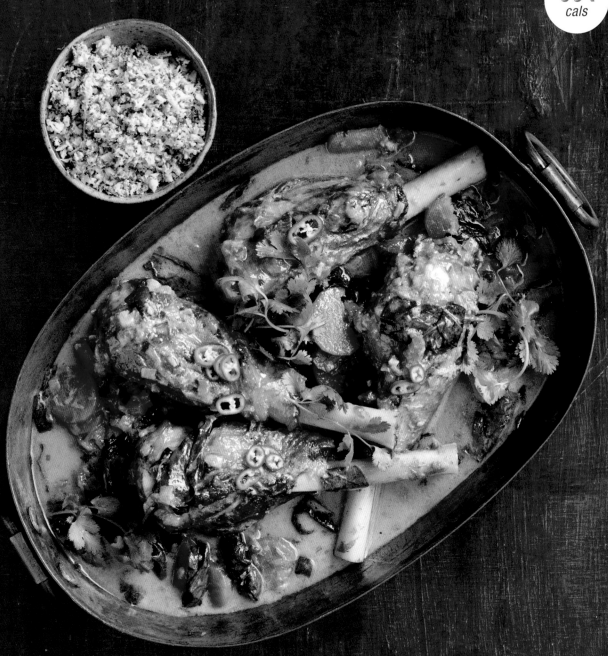

★★★★★ This was delicious. I started cooking at 5pm and we were eating by 7:45pm. Definitely recommend! **JESSMYKA**

ONE-PAN VEGETABLE
GNOCCHI

Take advantage of fresh seasonal ingredients with this light and luscious meat-free midweek meal.

SERVES 4 **PREP** 5 mins **COOK** 12 mins

500g pkt potato gnocchi
1 tbs olive oil, plus extra, to drizzle
2 tbs butter
250g cherry tomatoes, halved
2 garlic cloves, crushed
145g (1 cup) frozen shelled edamame
1 bunch asparagus, trimmed, sliced
30g parmesan, finely grated
Fresh basil leaves, to serve

1 Cook the gnocchi in a large saucepan of salted boiling water following packet directions, until tender. Drain. Transfer to a bowl and keep warm.

2 Melt the oil and butter in the same saucepan over medium-high heat until foaming and just light brown. Add the tomato. Cook, stirring, for 2-3 minutes or until the skins begin to blister. Add garlic. Cook for 30 seconds or until aromatic. Add edamame and asparagus. Cook, stirring, for 1-2 minutes or until tender-crisp.

3 Add the gnocchi to the pan and stir to coat. Season well. Add half the parmesan and stir to coat. Divide among serving bowls. Sprinkle with the remaining parmesan. Season with pepper. Drizzle with extra oil and top with basil leaves.

NON-FAST DAYS

Add a poached egg to each serve for a protein boost. 65 cals per serve.

NUTRITION (PER SERVE)

CALS	FAT	SAT FAT	PROTEIN	CARBS
415	20g	7g	9g	30g

★★★★★ *This is pretty great when looking for something quick and tasty. Next time I'll increase the vegie content by 50% – there's enough sauce and gnocchi to keep it tasty.* **HOTPOCKET**

● VEGETARIAN   ○ VEGAN   ○ GLUTEN FREE   ○ MAKE AHEAD   ○ FREEZABLE

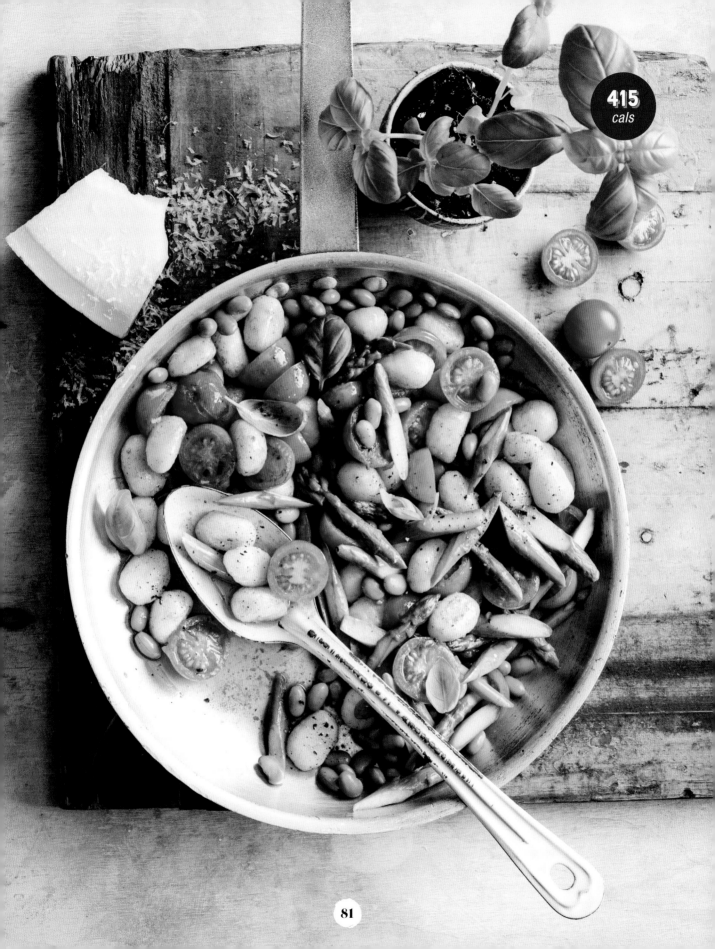

415
cals

TANDOORI PANEER WITH RAITA

This super-fast curry uses paneer, an Indian-style cheese that doesn't melt, to create a vego-friendly hearty meal.

SERVES 4 **PREP** 15 mins **COOK** 10 mins

2 tbs tandoori paste
130g (½ cup) Greek-style yoghurt
200g pkt paneer, cut into 2cm pieces
1½ tbs coconut oil
1 large red onion, halved, thinly sliced
1 large red capsicum, deseeded,
   thinly sliced
⅓ cup fresh mint leaves,
   finely chopped
250g pkt microwave brown, red and
   wild rice, cooked
120g baby spinach
1 Lebanese cucumber, halved,
   sliced diagonally
8 mini pappadums, microwaved
Lemon wedges, to serve (optional)

1 Combine the tandoori paste and 1 tbs yoghurt in a bowl. Add the paneer. Stir to coat.

2 Heat 1 tbs coconut oil in a non-stick frying pan over medium-high heat. Cook onion and capsicum, stirring occasionally, for 5 minutes or until softened. Add paneer mixture and remaining coconut oil. Cook, stirring, for 2 minutes. Add 2 tbs water and cook for a further minute or until golden and heated through.

3 Meanwhile, combine the mint and the remaining yoghurt in a bowl. Season.

4 Divide the rice, spinach, cucumber and paneer among serving plates. Serve with yoghurt raita, pappadums and lemon wedges, if using.

COOK'S NOTE

Paneer is a excellent source of fat-soluble vitamins A and D.

NUTRITION (PER SERVE)

CALS	FAT	SAT FAT	PROTEIN	CARBS
434	17.5g	11g	18.5g	35.5g

● VEGETARIAN   ○ VEGAN   ○ GLUTEN FREE   ○ MAKE AHEAD   ○ FREEZABLE

434
cals

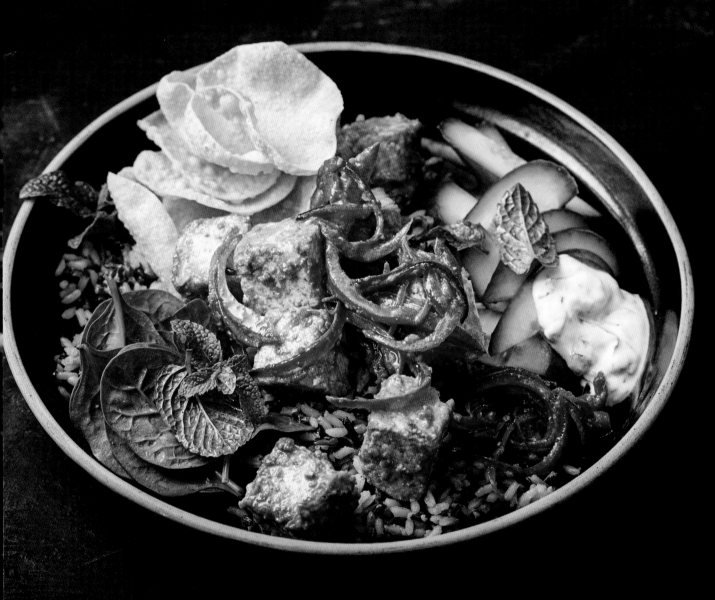

QUINOA-STUFFED
CAPSICUMS

A delicious quinoa and herb stuffing takes these roasted capsicums
to the next level, and is a good source of plant protein and fibre.

SERVES 4 **PREP** 15 mins **COOK** 55 mins

145g (¾ cup) tricoloured quinoa
1 lemon, rind finely grated, juiced
4 green shallots, thinly sliced
400g can red kidney beans,
    rinsed, drained
2 truss tomatoes, chopped
2 tbs chopped fresh coriander
2 tbs chopped fresh
    continental parsley
45g (¼ cup) pepitas
4 large mixed capsicums,
    halved lengthways, deseeded,
    membrane removed
55g (⅓ cup) cashews, soaked
    in cold water for 2 hours
1 tbs tahini
100g baby rocket leaves, to serve

1 Preheat oven to 200°C/180°C fan forced. Line a large baking tray with baking paper. Bring quinoa and 375ml (1½ cups) water to the boil in a saucepan over medium heat. Reduce heat to low. Cover and simmer for 12-15 minutes or until water is absorbed and quinoa is al dente. Remove from heat. Cool slightly.

2 Place quinoa, lemon rind, shallot, beans, tomato, coriander, parsley and pepitas in a large bowl. Season and stir to combine.

3 Stuff capsicum halves with quinoa mixture. Place on prepared tray. Spray with olive oil. Cover with foil. Bake for 20 minutes. Remove foil and bake for a further 15 minutes or until capsicums are tender and stuffing is golden.

4 Meanwhile, drain cashews. Place cashews, tahini, 60ml (¼ cup) water and 2 tsp lemon juice in a blender and blend until smooth.

5 Drizzle capsicums with cashew dressing and serve with baby rocket leaves.

NON-FAST DAYS

Add 1 medium
avocado, sliced,
to rocket leaves.
55 cals per serve.

NUTRITION (PER SERVE)

CALS	FAT	SAT FAT	PROTEIN	CARBS
381	15g	2g	16g	39g

● VEGETARIAN ● VEGAN ● GLUTEN FREE ● MAKE AHEAD ○ FREEZABLE

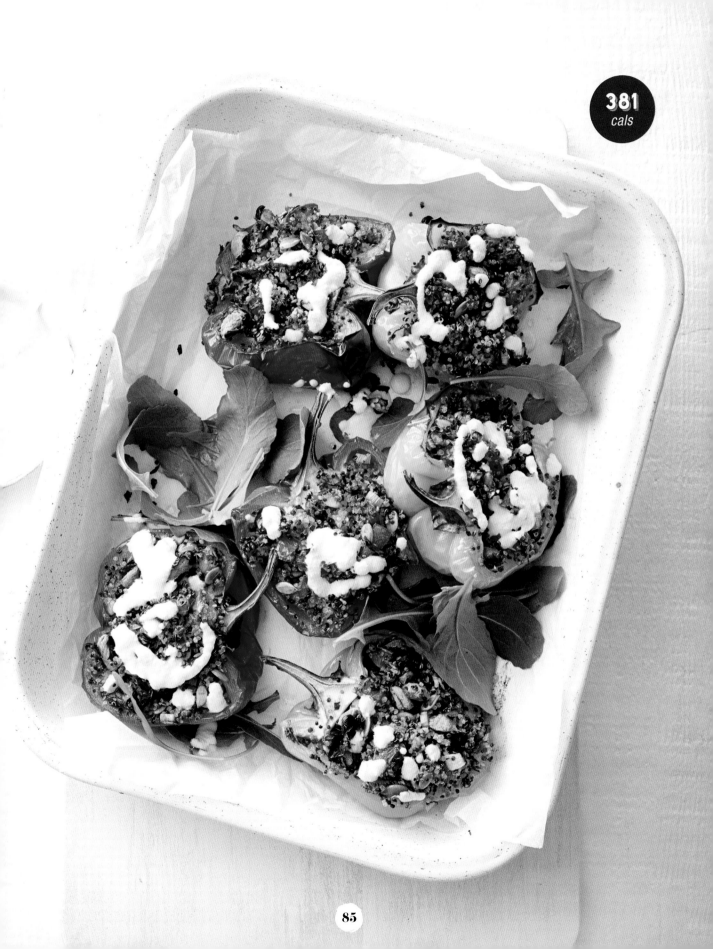

ONE-PAN SPAGHETTI

BOLOGNAISE

We've taken all of the flavour and removed all the stress (and most of the washing up) with this fast and easy version of a family favourite.

SERVES 6 **PREP** 5 mins **COOK** 20 mins

1 tbs extra virgin olive oil
500g lean pork and veal mince
2 tbs tomato paste
125ml (½ cup) red wine
400g jar bolognaise pasta sauce
2 large sprigs fresh rosemary
500ml (2 cups) chicken stock
375g pkt fresh fettuccine
Chopped fresh continental
  parsley, to serve
20g (¼ cup) grated parmesan,
  to serve

1 Heat the oil in a large, deep frying pan over high heat. Add the mince. Cook, breaking up any lumps with a wooden spoon, for 4 minutes or until it changes colour. Season well with salt.

2 Add the tomato paste and cook, stirring, for 1 minute. Add the wine. Simmer for 1-2 minutes or until nearly evaporated. Add the pasta sauce and rosemary. Simmer for 5 minutes or until reduced slightly.

3 Stir in the stock. Add the pasta and 250ml (1 cup) water. Cover and simmer for 2 minutes. Uncover and simmer, stirring occasionally, for a further 2-3 minutes or until the pasta is tender. Season with pepper. Serve sprinkled with parsley and parmesan.

NUTRITION (PER SERVE)

CALS	FAT	SAT FAT	PROTEIN	CARBS
467	16.8g	5.5g	31.8g	41.7g

★★★★★ *This was a super easy and super delicious weeknight meal – the whole family loved it. It tasted even better on the second day. Will definitely be making this one again, thank you!* **JAMIEANNE**

○ VEGETARIAN   ○ VEGAN   ○ GLUTEN FREE   ● MAKE AHEAD   ● FREEZABLE

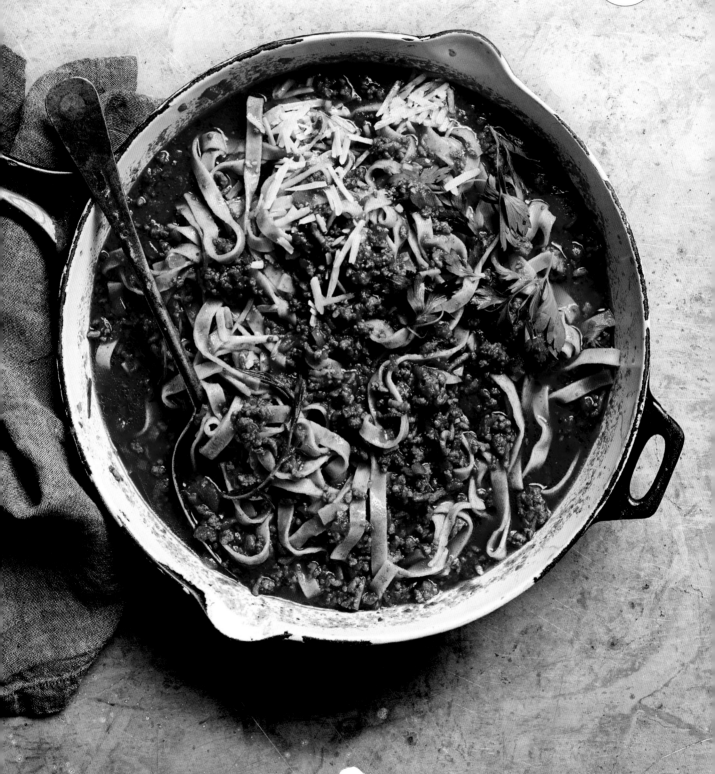

467
cals

FISH NACHOS WITH CABBAGE

Corn chips, fish and extra vegies combine to create a kid-friendly and gluten-free meal that's ready in under 20 minutes.

SERVES 4 **PREP** 15 mins **COOK** 5 mins

500g white fish fillets (such as flathead), cut into 4-5cm pieces
2-3 tsp gluten-free chipotle seasoning or Mexican chilli powder, to taste
1 tbs extra virgin olive oil
400g red cabbage
425g can black beans, rinsed, drained
200g cherry tomatoes, halved
3 green shallots, thinly sliced
1 tbs Greek-style yoghurt
1 large lime, rind finely grated, juiced, plus extra lime wedges, to serve
1 small avocado, mashed
⅓ cup fresh coriander leaves, chopped, plus extra to serve
50g gluten-free corn chips

1 Combine the fish, chipotle seasoning or chilli powder and 2 tsp oil in a bowl. Season.

2 Shred the cabbage in a food processor fitted with the slicing attachment. Transfer to a large bowl with the black beans, tomato, 2 shallots, yoghurt, lime rind, 2 tbs lime juice and the remaining oil. Season. Toss well to combine.

3 Heat a large non-stick frying pan over high heat. Cook the fish, turning, for 4 minutes or until just cooked through. Transfer to a plate.

4 Meanwhile, put the avocado, coriander, remaining shallot and 1 tbs remaining lime juice in a small bowl. Season and stir to combine.

5 Divide the cabbage mixture, fish, guacamole and corn chips among serving bowls. Scatter extra coriander over and serve with extra lime wedges.

COOK'S NOTE

Serve nachos sprinkled with 1 sliced red chilli for added heat.

NUTRITION (PER SERVE)

CALS	FAT	SAT FAT	PROTEIN	CARBS
409	16g	4g	36.5g	22.5g

○ VEGETARIAN   ○ VEGAN   ● GLUTEN FREE   ○ MAKE AHEAD   ○ FREEZABLE

409
cals

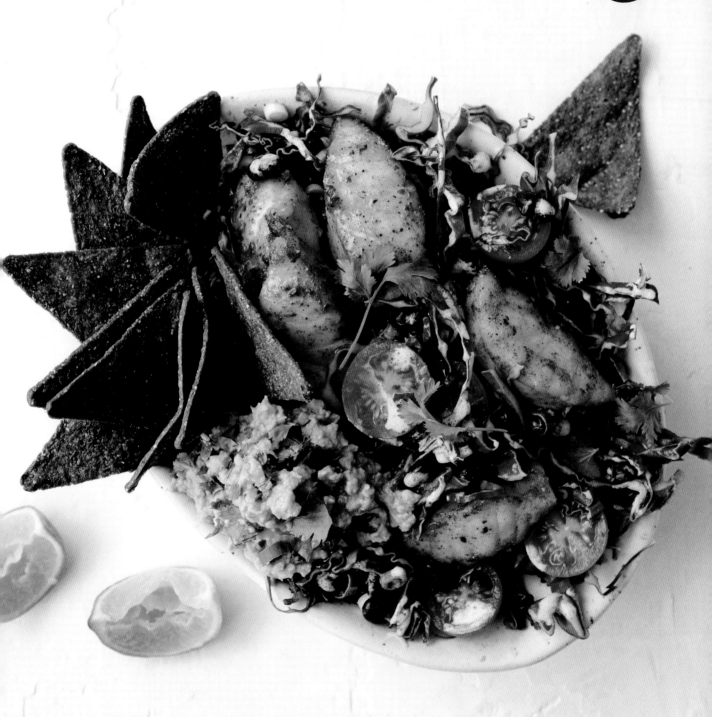

HEALTHIER CHICKEN
CACCIATORE

With a few clever tweaks, this Italian classic becomes better for you and easier, while still retaining its traditional flavours.

SERVES 6 **PREP** 25 mins **COOK** 1 hour 5 mins

6 (about 1.1kg) chicken thigh cutlets, skin removed
2 tbs olive oil
200g Swiss brown mushrooms, sliced
1 red onion, thinly sliced
4 ripe tomatoes, chopped
4 garlic cloves, chopped
1 red capsicum, deseeded, chopped
1 yellow capsicum, deseeded, chopped
1 carrot, peeled, chopped
125ml (½ cup) white wine
250ml (1 cup) gluten-free chicken stock
200g grape or cherry tomatoes
40g (¼ cup) pitted kalamata olives
2 tbs chopped fresh oregano leaves, plus extra sprigs, to serve

1 Season the chicken cutlets well. Heat 1 tbs olive oil in a large non-stick frying pan over medium-high heat. Cook the chicken for 2-3 minutes each side or until browned all over. Transfer to a plate.

2 Add the mushroom to the pan and cook, stirring, over medium heat for 3-4 minutes or until softened. Transfer to a bowl. Add the remaining 1 tbs oil to pan. Add the onion and cook, stirring, for 2-3 minutes or until just beginning to soften.

3 Add the chopped tomato and garlic. Cook, stirring, for 3-4 minutes, until softened. Add the capsicum and carrot and cook for 2 minutes. Add wine and simmer for 5 minutes or until liquid has reduced by half.

4 Return the chicken and mushroom to the pan. Add the stock, grape or cherry tomatoes, and the olives. Bring to the boil. Reduce the heat, cover and simmer for 20 minutes. Uncover and simmer for a further 20 minutes or until the liquid has reduced and sauce has thickened. Stir in the chopped oregano. Season.

5 Divide the chicken among serving bowls and scatter with extra oregano sprigs.

NON-FAST DAYS

Serve with 1 slice multigrain gluten-free bread per person. 93 cals per serve.

NUTRITION (PER SERVE)

CALS	FAT	SAT FAT	PROTEIN	CARBS
401	22g	5g	33g	9g

○ VEGETARIAN ○ VEGAN ● GLUTEN FREE ● MAKE AHEAD ● FREEZABLE

401
cals

★★★★★ *Beautiful, healthy dish that I've now made several times.* **KMCCARTNEY**

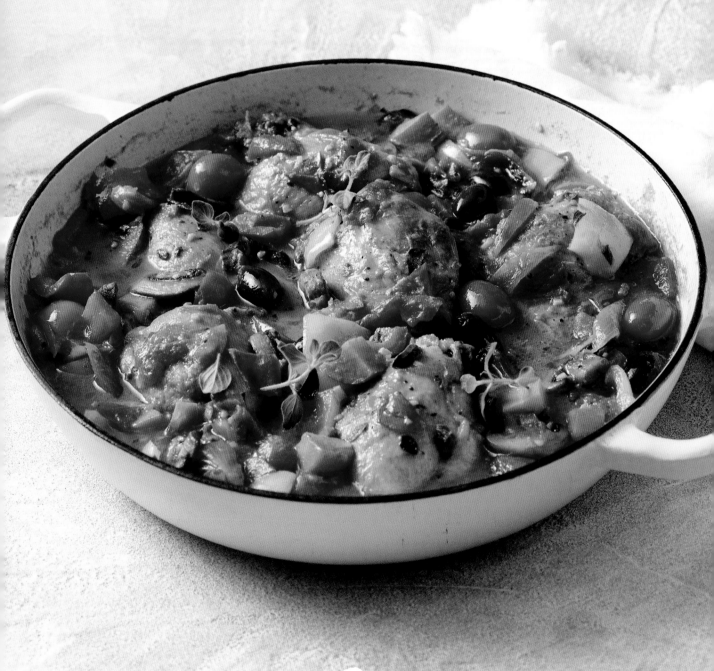

HARISSA CHICKEN & LENTIL BAKE

Packed full of flavour, this healthy tray bake has more than three serves of veg and the added protein of chicken and lentils.

SERVES 4 **PREP** 15 mins (+ 10 mins marinating) **COOK** 35 mins

3 small carrots, peeled, sliced diagonally

2 large red onions, cut into thin wedges

1 tbs chopped fresh rosemary leaves

1 tbs extra virgin olive oil

2 tsp harissa paste

1 lemon, rind zested, juiced

1 garlic clove, crushed

8 (about 500g) chicken tenderloins, trimmed

400g can no-added-salt brown lentils, rinsed, drained

80g trimmed kale leaves, torn

160ml (⅔ cup) salt-reduced gluten-free chicken stock

90g (⅓ cup) labneh, drained

1 Preheat oven to 200°C/180°C fan forced. Line a large baking dish or tray with baking paper. Place the carrot, onion and rosemary in prepared dish and drizzle with the oil. Bake for 15-20 minutes or until light golden and tender.

2 Meanwhile, combine the harissa, 1 tbs lemon juice and garlic in a shallow dish. Add the chicken and turn to coat. Set aside for 10 minutes to marinate.

3 Place the lentils, kale and stock in the dish with the carrot mixture and stir to combine. Top with the chicken. Bake for a further 10-15 minutes or until chicken is cooked through. Top with labneh and a little lemon zest. Season and serve.

NON-FAST DAYS

Double the amount of labneh in this dish for extra creaminess. 23 cals per serve.

NUTRITION (PER SERVE)

CALS	FAT	SAT FAT	PROTEIN	CARBS
341	9.5g	2.5g	37.5g	20g

★★★★★ *Loved by the whole family – even my dad who is a self-confessed kale and lentil hater liked it. Simple, tasty and minimal washing up. Win, win, win!* **IMOGENR**

○ VEGETARIAN ○ VEGAN ● GLUTEN FREE ○ MAKE AHEAD ○ FREEZABLE

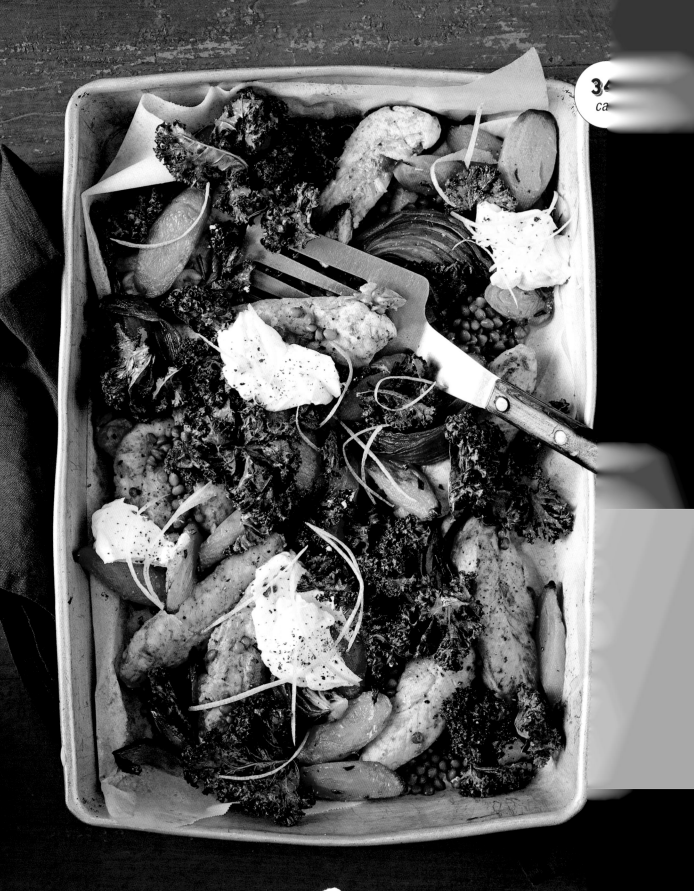

MEXICAN TURMERIC FISH

Accompanied by a spicy mango salsa, this fish dish is full of nutrient-dense ingredients, including black beans and kale.

SERVES 4 **PREP** 15 mins **COOK** 10 mins

1 mango, cheeks removed, flesh chopped
¼ cup chopped fresh coriander, plus extra leaves, to serve
1 tbs fresh lime juice
2 fresh long red chillies, deseeded, finely chopped
4 x 125g firm white fish fillets
1 tsp ground turmeric
1 tbs extra virgin olive oil
2 garlic cloves, crushed
400g can black beans, rinsed, drained
150g trimmed kale, chopped
300g (2 cups) cooked quinoa, warmed

1 Combine the mango, coriander, lime juice and half the chilli in a bowl. Set aside. Dust the fish fillets with the turmeric to lightly coat.

2 Heat 2 tsp oil in a large non-stick frying pan or wok over medium-high heat. Cook the garlic and remaining chilli, stirring, for 1 minute or until aromatic. Add the black beans and cook, stirring, for 1 minute or until warmed through. Add the kale and use tongs to toss for 2 minutes or until just wilted. Cover to keep warm.

3 Heat the remaining 2 tsp oil in a large non-stick frying pan over medium-high heat. Cook the fish for 2-3 minutes each side or until golden and cooked through.

4 Divide the quinoa among serving bowls. Top with the black bean mixture, fish and mango salsa. Serve with extra coriander scattered on top.

COOK'S NOTE

You can swap the mango with 2 small fresh nectarines or peaches.

NUTRITION (PER SERVE)

CALS	FAT	SAT FAT	PROTEIN	CARBS
359	9g	2g	34g	31g

★★★★★ *This was a great recipe – I added in avocado to the salsa. This will be one we will regularly make from now on.* **MIHELIC**

○ VEGETARIAN   ○ VEGAN   ● GLUTEN FREE   ○ MAKE AHEAD   ○ FREEZABLE

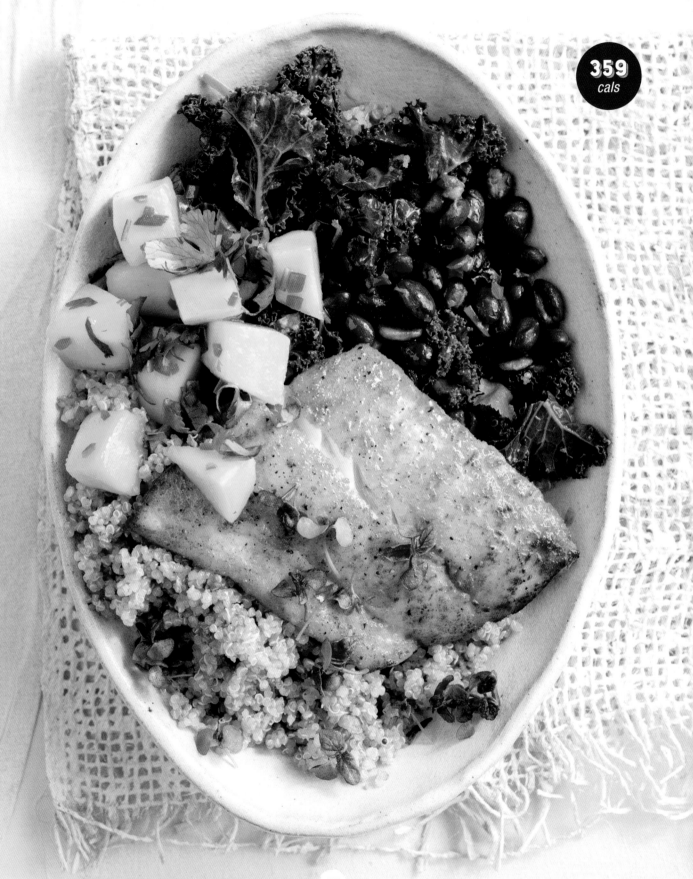

359
cals

FRYING-PAN ZUCCHINI
BOLOGNAISE

Increase your vegie count with this gluten-free twist on everyone's favourite family dinner – and it's on the table in less than half an hour too!

SERVES 4   **PREP** 10 mins   **COOK** 15 mins

1 brown onion, quartered
1 carrot, peeled, quartered
2 garlic cloves, peeled
2 tbs extra virgin olive oil
1½ tsp dried oregano leaves
500g lean beef mince
1 tbs tomato paste
500g jar gluten-free tomato
   or bolognaise pasta sauce
2 x 250g pkt zucchini noodles
100g (1 cup) coarsely grated
   mozzarella
Fresh oregano leaves, to serve
   (optional)

1 Place onion, carrot and garlic in a food processor. Process until finely chopped. Heat 1 tbs oil in a deep, ovenproof frying pan over high heat. Add onion mixture and 1 tsp dried oregano. Cook, stirring occasionally, for 3 minutes or until softened.

2 Add the beef and remaining oil. Cook, breaking up any lumps with a wooden spoon, for 3 minutes or until browned. Stir in tomato paste for 1 minute or until combined.

3 Stir in the pasta sauce. Cook, covered, for 2 minutes. Gently stir in the zucchini noodles. Cook, covered, for a further 2 minutes or until just tender. Remove the pan from heat.

4 Preheat the oven grill to high. Sprinkle bolognaise with mozzarella and remaining dried oregano. Grill for 2-3 minutes or until cheese is golden and melted. Top with fresh oregano, if using.

COOK'S NOTE

You can add ½ tsp dried red chilli flakes in step 1 for a spicy version of this recipe.

NUTRITION (PER SERVE)

CALS	FAT	SAT FAT	PROTEIN	CARBS
430	22.5g	7.5g	38.5g	15.5g

○ VEGETARIAN   ○ VEGAN   ● GLUTEN FREE   ● MAKE AHEAD   ● FREEZABLE

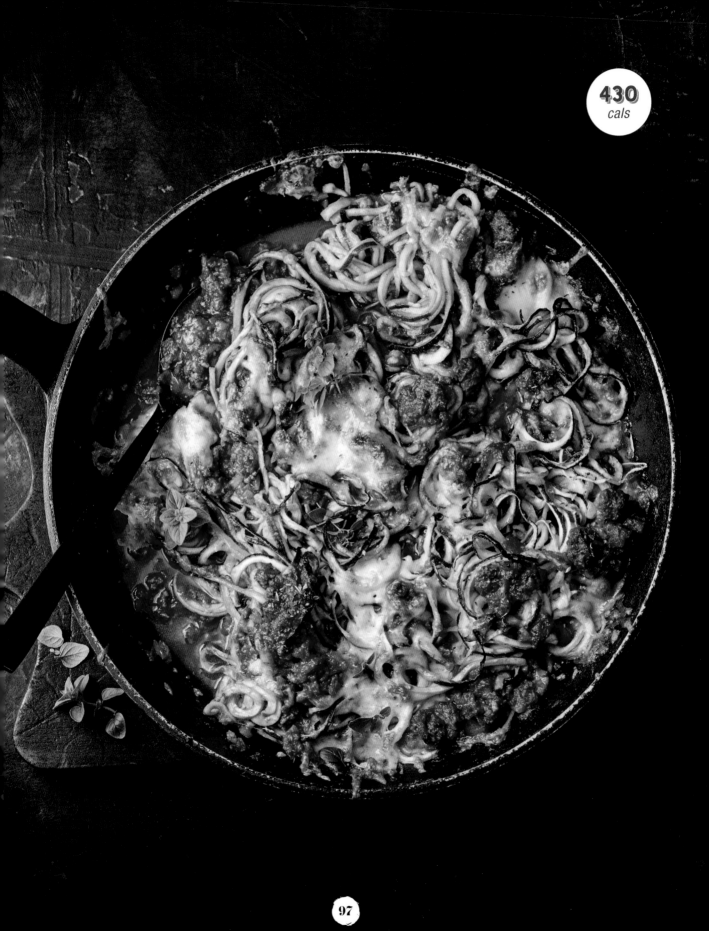

430
cals

SUMAC CHICKEN WITH CHICKPEAS

This spiced chicken salad is served with pita bread and baba ghanoush to create a refreshing mix of Middle Eastern flavours.

SERVES 4 **PREP** 15 mins (+ 10 mins marinating) **COOK** 10 mins

1 garlic clove, crushed
1 tsp sumac
1 tsp ground cumin
1 tsp extra virgin olive oil
1½ tbs fresh lemon juice
500g chicken tenderloins
400g can chickpeas, rinsed, drained
4 green shallots, thinly sliced
250g cherry tomatoes, halved
75g trimmed English spinach, chopped
1 tbs sunflower seeds, lightly toasted
2 tbs baba ghanoush, to serve
2 small (31g each) wholemeal pita pockets, halved, cut into wedges

1 Combine garlic, sumac, cumin, oil and 1 tbs of the lemon juice in a shallow dish. Add the chicken and turn to coat. Cover and set aside for 10 minutes to marinate.

2 Meanwhile, combine chickpeas, shallot, tomato, spinach, sunflower seeds and remaining 2 tsp lemon juice in a large bowl.

3 Preheat a chargrill or barbecue grill on medium-high. Drain chicken, discard excess marinade. Lightly spray with olive oil. Cook, turning, for 3 minutes each side or until just cooked through and lightly charred.

4 Serve chicken with the chickpea salad, baba ghanoush and accompanied by pita bread.

NON-FAST DAYS

Crumble 100g feta over and double the quantity of pita bread. 113 cals per serve.

NUTRITION (PER SERVE)

CALS	FAT	SAT FAT	PROTEIN	CARBS
326	7g	1g	36g	24g

○ VEGETARIAN   ○ VEGAN   ○ GLUTEN FREE   ○ MAKE AHEAD   ○ FREEZABLE

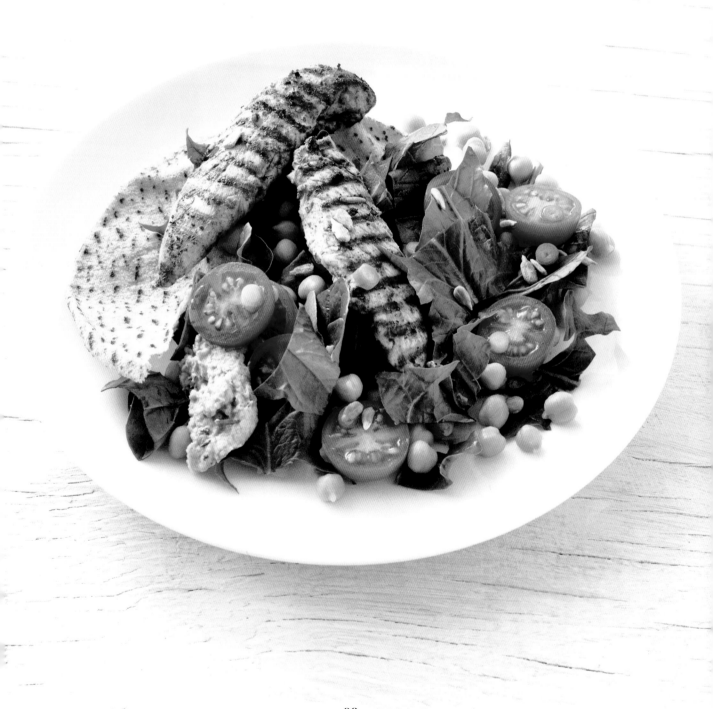

BARLEY, CHICKPEA & EGGPLANT

This vegie casserole is ready in under an hour and is topped with parsley pesto for a fresh hit of herbs.

SERVES 4 **PREP** 20 mins **COOK** 40 mins

1½ tbs extra virgin olive oil
1 small (about 350g) eggplant, cut into 2cm pieces
1 large red onion, finely chopped
2 large celery sticks, coarsely chopped
3 garlic cloves, thinly sliced
1 lemon, rind finely grated, juiced
150g (¾ cup) pearl barley, rinsed, drained
250ml (1 cup) homemade or reduced-salt vegetable stock
400g can chickpeas, rinsed, drained
2 zucchini, coarsely chopped
250g cherry tomatoes, halved
½ cup firmly packed fresh continental parsley leaves, plus extra leaves, to serve
20g (¼ cup) finely grated parmesan

1 Heat 2 tsp of oil in a large non-stick saucepan over high heat. Add the eggplant. Cook, stirring, for 2-3 minutes or until golden. Transfer to a plate and set aside.

2 Reduce heat to medium. Add 1 tsp of remaining oil, onion and celery. Cook, stirring, for 5 minutes or until vegetables soften. Add the garlic and lemon rind. Stir for 1 minute or until aromatic. Add the barley, stock and 500ml (2 cups) water. Bring to the boil. Reduce heat. Cover and simmer, stirring occasionally, for 25 minutes or until liquid has almost evaporated and the barley is al dente. Add the chickpeas, zucchini, tomato and eggplant. Simmer for 5 minutes or until zucchini is tender. Season.

3 Meanwhile, place parsley, parmesan, 1 tbs lemon juice, remaining oil and 2 tsp water in a small food processor. Process until smooth. Season.

4 Top the casserole with a dollop of parsley pesto and extra parsley leaves. Serve remaining pesto on the side.

NON-FAST DAYS

Top casserole with 60g crumbled feta. 42 cals per serve.

NUTRITION (PER SERVE)

CALS	FAT	SAT FAT	PROTEIN	CARBS
333	11g	2.5g	12g	39g

● VEGETARIAN ○ VEGAN ○ GLUTEN FREE ● MAKE AHEAD ○ FREEZABLE

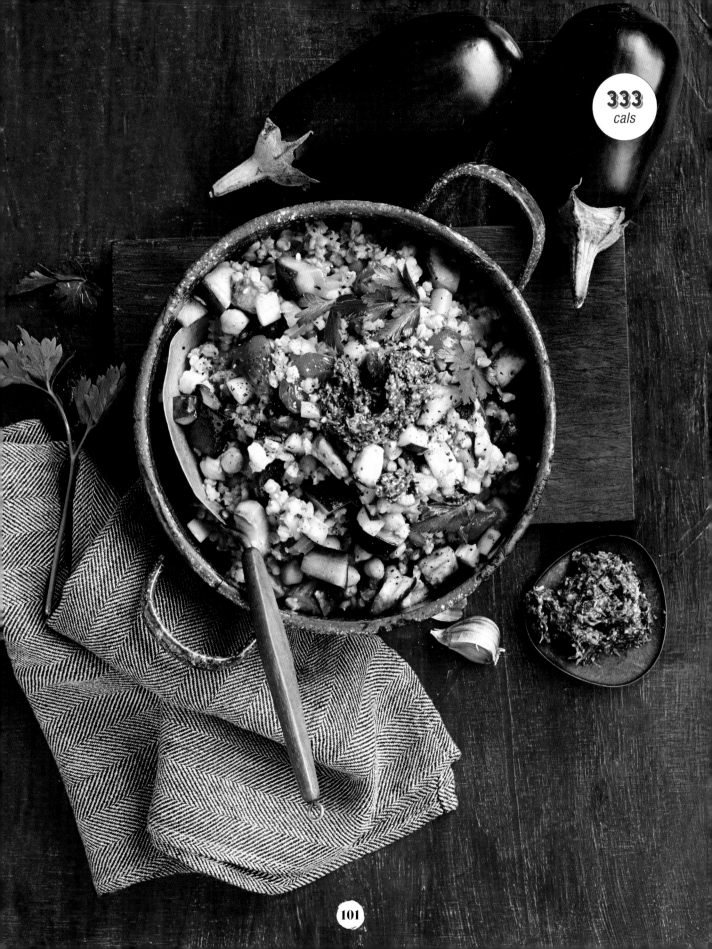

333
cals

LAMB, CHICKPEA & PUMPKIN BAKE

This hearty bake is easy to throw together and uses pumpkin instead of lasagne noodles for a vegie-filled meal.

SERVES 6 **PREP** 20 mins (+ 10 mins cooling) **COOK** 1 hour 5 mins

1.2kg butternut pumpkin, peeled, deseeded, thinly sliced

3 tsp ground cumin

1 tsp olive oil

1 large red onion, finely chopped

4 celery sticks, trimmed, finely chopped

2 garlic cloves, crushed

1 tsp ground cinnamon

500g lean lamb mince

400g can diced tomatoes

400g can no-added-salt chickpeas, rinsed and drained

1 zucchini, finely chopped

240g (1 cup) fresh ricotta

1 egg

130g (½ cup) natural yoghurt

¼ cup chopped fresh continental parsley

260g cherry truss tomatoes

Baby French kale or rocket leaves, to serve

1 Preheat the oven to 200°C/180°C fan forced. Line 2 baking trays with baking paper. Place pumpkin on trays, spray with oil and sprinkle with half the cumin. Bake, swapping trays halfway, for 25-30 minutes or until golden and tender.

2 Meanwhile, heat the olive oil in a large saucepan over medium heat. Cook the onion and celery, stirring occasionally, for 7-8 minutes or until softened. Add the garlic, cinnamon and remaining cumin and cook, stirring, for 1 minute or until aromatic.

3 Add the mince and cook, breaking up any lumps with a wooden spoon, for 5 minutes or until browned. Add the diced tomato, chickpeas, zucchini and 185ml (¾ cup) water, and bring to the boil. Reduce the heat to low and simmer, stirring occasionally, for 20 minutes or until thick.

4 Combine the ricotta, egg, yoghurt and parsley in a bowl. Season. Lightly spray a 2L (8 cup) baking dish with oil. Spread half the mince mixture over the base of the prepared dish. Top with half the pumpkin. Repeat with another layer of mince mixture and pumpkin, then carefully spread the ricotta sauce over the top. Bake for 15 minutes.

5 Line a baking tray with baking paper, place the truss tomatoes on it and add to the oven with the bake. Bake for a further 15 minutes or until the bake is golden and bubbling and the tomatoes are just softened. Set the bake aside for 10 minutes to cool slightly. Top with the tomatoes and kale or rocket to serve.

NUTRITION (PER SERVE)

CALS	FAT	SAT FAT	PROTEIN	CARBS
354	14g	5g	30g	22g

○ VEGETARIAN   ○ VEGAN   ● GLUTEN FREE   ● MAKE AHEAD   ○ FREEZABLE

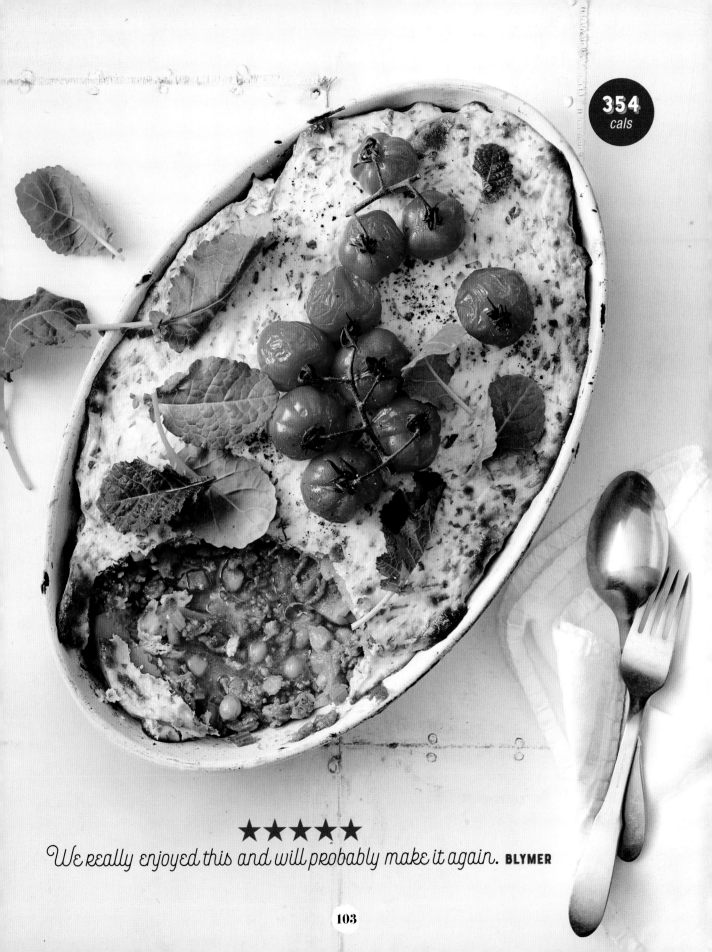

354 cals

★★★★★
We really enjoyed this and will probably make it again. BLYMER

COCONUT CHICKPEA
CURRY

Packed full of flavoursome ingredients, this coconut curry ticks all the nutrition boxes, and includes a hearty side of broccoli rice.

SERVES 4   **PREP** 20 mins (+ overnight soaking)   **COOK** 1 hour 10 mins

210g (1 cup) dried chickpeas
1 large red onion, chopped
3 garlic cloves, chopped
3cm-piece ginger, peeled, chopped
2 fresh long green chillies, chopped, plus sliced chilli, extra, to serve
1 tsp garam masala
2 tsp ground cumin
2 tsp macadamia oil
2 vine-ripened tomatoes, chopped
250ml (1 cup) gluten-free salt-reduced vegetable stock
125ml (½ cup) light coconut milk
300g peeled pumpkin, chopped
200g green beans, cut into 4cm lengths
1½ limes, cut into wedges
600g broccoli, coarsely chopped
Fresh coriander sprigs, to serve

1 Soak the chickpeas in a large bowl of water overnight. Drain. Place the chickpeas in a large saucepan and cover with cold water. Bring to the boil, then reduce the heat to low and simmer for 30-40 minutes or until tender. Drain. Set aside.

2 Process onion, garlic, ginger, chilli, garam masala and cumin in a small food processor until a thick paste forms. Heat macadamia oil in a large saucepan or wok over medium heat. Add the paste and stir for 1-2 minutes or until aromatic. Add tomato and stir for 1 minute.

3 Add the stock, coconut milk, cooked chickpeas and pumpkin to the pan and bring to the boil. Reduce heat to low, cover and simmer for 20 minutes. Add the beans, cover and simmer for 5 minutes or until the vegies are tender. Squeeze in a little lime juice.

4 Meanwhile, process the broccoli, in batches, in a food processor until coarse crumbs form. Steam or microwave the broccoli rice until just tender. Drain.

5 Serve the curry on the broccoli rice. Top with coriander and extra chilli. Serve with the remaining lime wedges.

NUTRITION (PER SERVE)

CALS	FAT	SAT FAT	PROTEIN	CARBS
363	7g	3g	25g	38g

● VEGETARIAN   ● VEGAN   ● GLUTEN FREE   ● MAKE AHEAD   ○ FREEZABLE

363
cals

★★★★★ *Have cooked this twice now with and without the broccoli rice and every last bit has been eaten!* **DINPIP4**

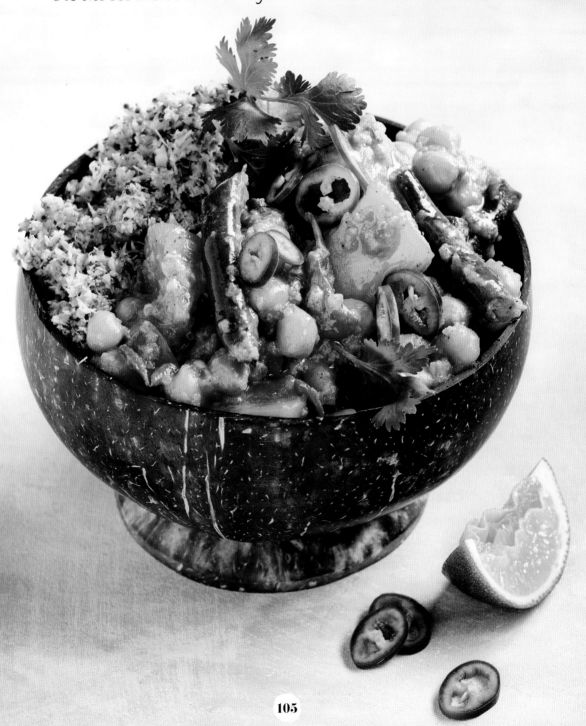

PORK & PUMPKIN WITH
CHIMICHURRI

The tangy herb and garlic Argentine sauce provides the ideal balance for lean and healthy pork fillets and mouth-watering roast pumpkin.

SERVES 4 **PREP** 15 mins **COOK** 50 mins

1.2kg kent pumpkin, skin on, cut into thin wedges
500g lean pork fillet
45g (¼ cup) smoked almonds, chopped
40g baby rocket

CHIMICHURRI
1 fresh long red chilli, chopped
2 garlic cloves, peeled
1 cup fresh coriander stems and leaves
⅓ cup fresh continental parsley leaves
½ cup fresh mint leaves
60ml (¼ cup) red wine vinegar
2 tsp pomegranate molasses (optional)
2 tbs olive oil

1 Preheat the oven to 220°C/200°C fan forced. Line 2 large baking trays with baking paper. Place pumpkin in a single layer on prepared trays. Spray with oil. Season. Bake for 35-40 minutes or until golden and tender.

2 Spray pork with oil and season well. Heat a frying pan over medium-high heat. Cook the pork for 4-5 minutes each side or until cooked to your liking. Transfer to a plate. Cover loosely with foil to keep warm and set aside to rest.

3 To make the chimichurri, place the chilli, garlic, coriander, parsley, mint, vinegar and molasses, if using, in a food processor. Process until finely chopped. Transfer to a small bowl and stir in the olive oil. Season well.

4 Thickly slice the pork. Arrange with the pumpkin wedges on a large serving platter. Scatter with the almonds and rocket. Drizzle with the chimichurri sauce.

NON-FAST DAYS

Add ½ cup steamed brown rice per person. 138 cals per serve.

NUTRITION (PER SERVE)

CALS	FAT	SAT FAT	PROTEIN	CARBS
404	20g	3g	35g	15g

○ VEGETARIAN ○ VEGAN ● GLUTEN FREE ● MAKE AHEAD ○ FREEZABLE

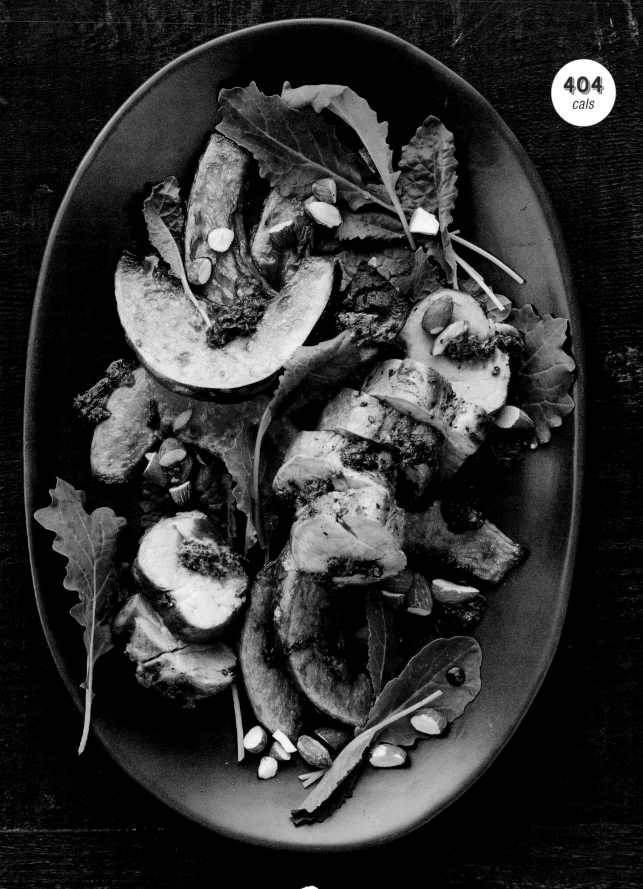

STIR-FRY WITH CHICKEN & VEGIES

On the table in 35 minutes, this vegie-laden noodle dish will please all the members of the family.

SERVES 4 **PREP** 20 mins **COOK** 15 mins

100g dried rice vermicelli noodles
2 tbs salt-reduced gluten-free tamari
1 tbs fresh lime juice
1 tsp brown sugar
500g chicken breast fillets, thinly sliced
1 red onion, cut into thin wedges
1 large carrot, halved, thinly sliced
1 fresh long red chilli, finely chopped
1 lemongrass stalk, pale section only, finely chopped
2 tsp finely grated fresh ginger
2 garlic cloves, finely chopped
1 large red capsicum, deseeded, thinly sliced
200g sugar snap peas, cut in half lengthways
250g zucchini noodles
Fresh basil leaves, to serve

1 Place the noodles in a large heatproof bowl. Cover with boiling water and set aside to soak for 5 minutes or until tender. Drain and set aside.

2 Combine the tamari, lime juice and sugar in a small bowl, stirring to dissolve the sugar. Set aside.

3 Spray a large wok with oil and heat over high heat. Stir-fry the chicken, in 2 batches, for 2-3 minutes each batch or until golden. Transfer to a plate.

4 Spray the wok with a little more oil. Add the onion and carrot and stir-fry for 2 minutes. Add the chilli, lemongrass, ginger and garlic and stir-fry for 1 minute or until aromatic. Add the capsicum, peas and 2 tbs water and stir-fry for 1 minute. Add the zucchini and vermicelli noodles and stir-fry for 1-2 minutes or until the vegetables are nearly tender.

5 Add the sauce mixture and the chicken to the wok. Stir-fry for 1-2 minutes or until heated through. Serve topped with fresh basil leaves.

NON-FAST DAYS

For a protein boost, increase chicken to 600g and sprinkle stir-fry with ¼ cup chopped unsalted cashew nuts. 72 cals per serve.

NUTRITION (PER SERVE)

CALS	FAT	SAT FAT	PROTEIN	CARBS
321	5.3g	1g	34.3g	29.5g

○ VEGETARIAN ○ VEGAN ● **GLUTEN FREE** ○ MAKE AHEAD ○ FREEZABLE

321
cals

★★★★★ *Delicious and easy. I left the seeds in my chilli when I sliced it and it added a nice zing. I also think coriander would go well with the rest of the ingredients.* **PAMMEO5**

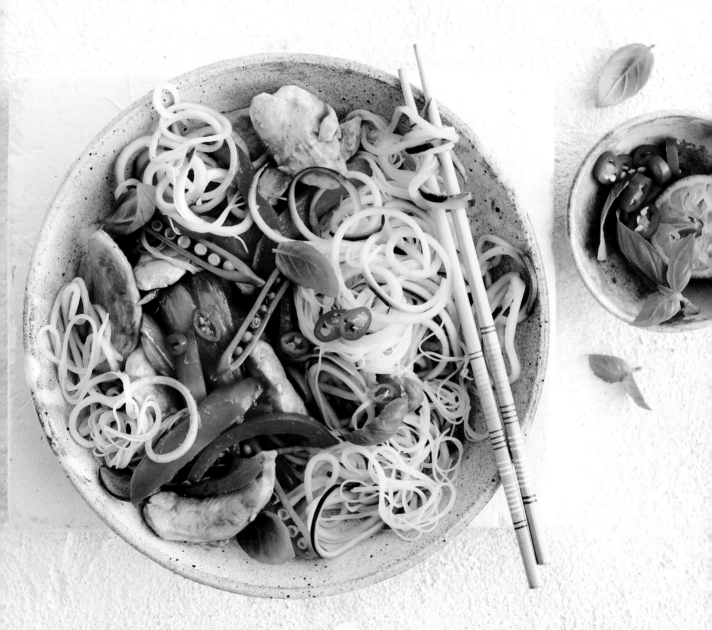

SALMON & PAPAYA
TACOS

Topped with a fruity salsa, these fresh-flavoured tacos turn a midweek meal into a Mexican-style fiesta.

SERVES 4 **PREP** 20 mins **COOK** 10 mins

2 (160g each) skinless salmon fillets
1½ tsp Mexican chilli powder
1 tsp ground cumin
1 tsp olive oil
2 red capsicums, deseeded, thinly sliced
60g (¼ cup) no-fat Greek-style yoghurt
½ tsp Sriracha chilli sauce
8 x 28g gluten-free corn tortillas, warmed
Fresh coriander leaves, to serve
Lime wedges, to serve

PAPAYA SALSA
300g papaya, peeled, cut into 1cm pieces
½ small avocado, cut into 1cm pieces
½ cup chopped fresh coriander leaves
1 large lime, rind finely grated, juiced
2 green shallots, finely chopped
1 fresh long green chilli, deseeded, finely chopped

1 Place the salmon in a bowl. Sprinkle with the chilli powder and cumin. Season well. Toss to coat.

2 For the papaya salsa, combine all the ingredients in a bowl. Season. Set aside to develop the flavours.

3 Heat the oil in a large non-stick frying pan over medium heat. Add the salmon and capsicum. Cook, stirring the capsicum occasionally, and turning salmon once, for 6 minutes or until the salmon is almost cooked through.

4 Meanwhile, place the yoghurt in a small bowl and swirl the chilli sauce through.

5 Flake the salmon into pieces. Fill tortillas with capsicum, salmon and salsa. Dollop with chilli yoghurt, sprinkle with coriander and serve with lime wedges.

COOK'S NOTE

For crispy tortillas, spray with olive oil spray and bake in a 180°C/200°C fan forced oven for 5 minutes.

NUTRITION (PER SERVE)

CALS	FAT	SAT FAT	PROTEIN	CARBS
478	21g	5g	26g	43g

○ VEGETARIAN ○ VEGAN ● GLUTEN FREE ○ MAKE AHEAD ○ FREEZABLE

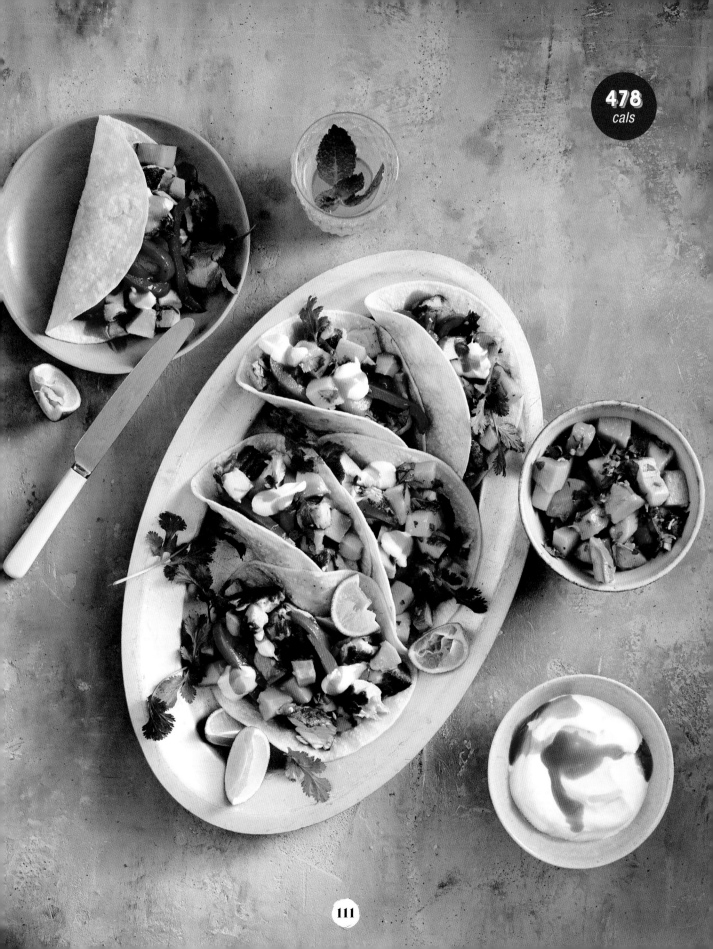

478
cals

SPICED 'RICE'
LAMB LEG

The spiced cauliflower rice makes a wonderful low-carb substitute for white rice, and absorbs all the delicious flavours from this dish.

SERVES 6 **PREP** 20 mins (+ 4 hours marinating) **COOK** 5 hours

1.6kg leg of lamb, bone in,
　visible fat trimmed
90g (⅓ cup) natural yoghurt
1 tsp ground coriander
3 tsp ground cumin
2 tsp ground turmeric
3 garlic cloves, crushed
1 large cauliflower, cut into florets
1 tbs extra virgin olive oil
1 large brown onion, thinly sliced
2 tsp brown mustard seeds
12 fresh curry leaves
300g green beans, trimmed, halved
　lengthways, steamed
2 tbs chopped fresh coriander
2 tbs chopped fresh
　continental parsley
Lemon juice, to taste
Fried curry leaves, to serve (optional)

1 Score the lamb at 2cm intervals. Combine yoghurt, ground coriander, 1 tsp cumin, 1 tsp turmeric and 1 garlic clove in a glass dish. Add lamb. Turn to coat, rubbing into scores. Cover. Place in fridge for 4 hours to marinate.

2 Preheat oven to 160°C/140°C fan forced. Transfer the lamb to a roasting pan. Add 500ml (2 cups) water to pan. Cover the lamb with baking paper. Cover the pan with foil. Roast for 5 hours, removing foil and paper for the last 30 minutes of cooking, or until lamb is tender. Set aside to rest for 10 minutes.

3 Meanwhile, process the cauliflower in batches in a food processor until coarsely chopped. Heat oil in a wok over high heat. Stir fry the onion for 2-3 minutes or until golden. Stir fry the mustard seeds, curry leaves and remaining cumin, turmeric and garlic for 30 seconds. Stir fry the cauliflower for 3-4 minutes or until tender. Stir fry the beans until combined. Stir in herbs and juice to taste.

4 Serve the cauliflower rice mixture with the lamb and fried curry leaves, if using.

NON-FAST DAYS

Cut 700g baby potatoes in half and toss with 2 tsp olive oil. Roast for 1 hour. 89 cals per serve.

NUTRITION (PER SERVE)

CALS	FAT	SAT FAT	PROTEIN	CARBS
313	14g	5g	36g	6g

○ VEGETARIAN　○ VEGAN　● GLUTEN FREE　○ MAKE AHEAD　○ FREEZABLE

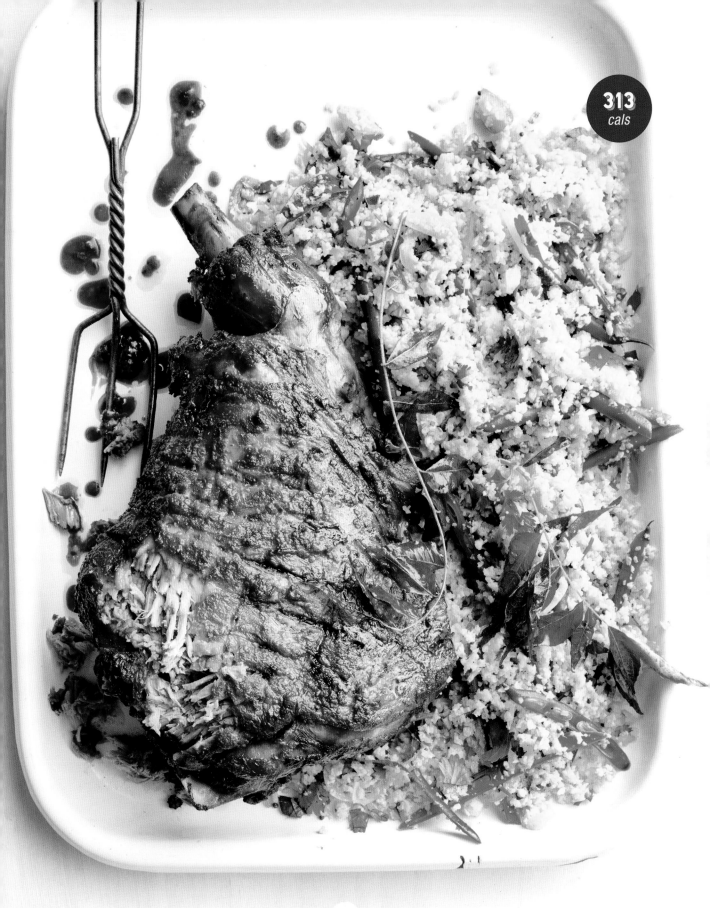

313
cals

CHICKEN & VEGIES WITH BARLEY

Chargrilled vegies provide a great flavour base for the grilled chicken fillets in this dish, served with barley for added heartiness.

SERVES 4 **PREP** 15 mins **COOK** 25 mins

165g (¾ cup) pearl barley
1 tbs olive oil
1 red onion, finely chopped
2 garlic cloves, crushed
1 tsp ground cumin
400g can no-added-salt chickpeas, rinsed, drained
80ml (⅓ cup) salt-reduced chicken stock
2 tbs fresh lemon juice
1 eggplant, trimmed, cut into 1cm slices
2 capsicums, deseeded, cut into thin wedges
2 zucchini, trimmed, cut into 1cm slices
2 (200g each) chicken breast fillets
Mixed salad leaves, including micro leaves (optional), to serve

1 Cook the barley in a large saucepan of boiling water for 25 minutes or until al dente. Drain.

2 Meanwhile, heat 2 tsp oil in a saucepan over medium heat. Add the onion and cook, stirring, for 3-4 minutes or until soft. Add the garlic and cumin and cook, stirring, for 1 minute or until aromatic. Add the chickpeas and stock to the pan and simmer for 2 minutes. Remove from the heat. Use a potato masher to mash the chickpeas, keeping some texture. Stir through 1 tbs lemon juice. Season. Cover to keep warm and set aside.

3 Heat a large chargrill pan over medium-high heat. Spray the eggplant, capsicum, zucchini and chicken lightly with olive oil. Cook the chicken for 4-5 minutes each side or until golden and cooked through. Cook the vegetables for 2 minutes each side or until lightly charred and tender.

4 Combine remaining lemon juice and olive oil. Slice the chicken. Divide the barley, chargrilled vegetables, chicken and salad leaves among bowls. Drizzle with the dressing and top with smashed chickpeas and micro leaves, if using.

COOK'S NOTE

Serve with ½ grilled corncob per person as a side dish. 71 cals each.

NUTRITION (PER SERVE)

CALS	FAT	SAT FAT	PROTEIN	CARBS
433	10g	2g	35g	43g

○ VEGETARIAN ○ VEGAN ○ GLUTEN FREE ○ MAKE AHEAD ○ FREEZABLE

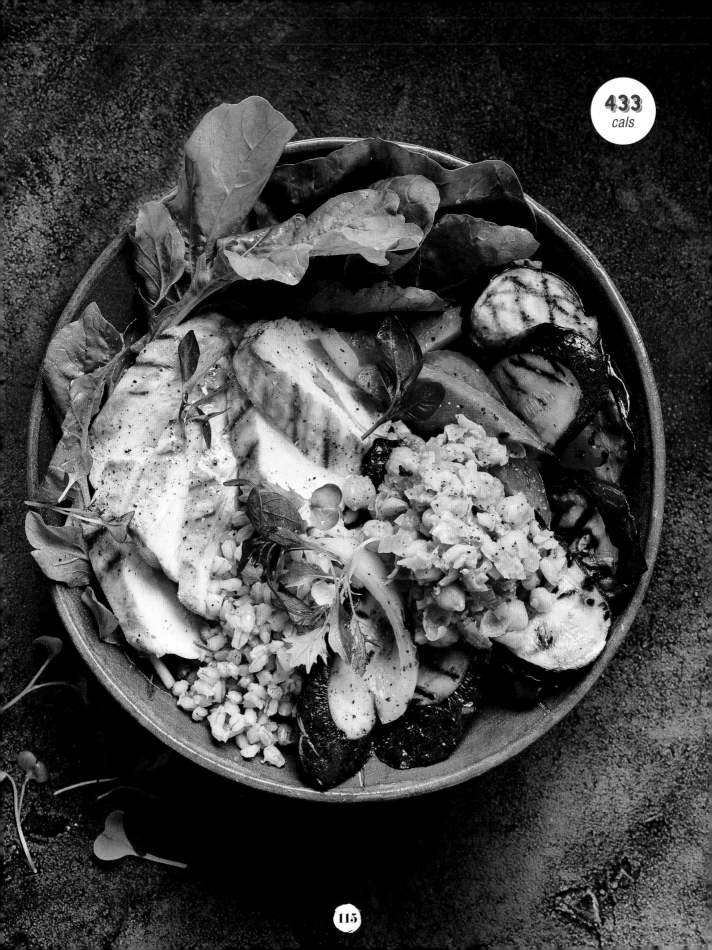

433
cals

ONE-TRAY SPICED POTATO &

SALMON

With turmeric, chilli, mustard seeds and coriander, this vibrantly coloured salmon and vegetable tray bake will be a new dinner staple.

SERVES 4 **PREP** 15 mins **COOK** 45 mins

1 tsp ground coriander
½ tsp ground turmeric
2 tsp mustard seeds
½ tsp ground chilli
500g baby potatoes, halved
230g (1½ cups) frozen green peas
1 bunch broccolini, halved
175g mini capsicums
250g cherry truss tomatoes
4 x 120g skinless salmon fillets
90g (⅓ cup) natural yoghurt
1 tbs fresh lime juice, plus extra
   wedges, to serve
2 tbs chopped fresh coriander leaves,
   plus extra sprigs, to serve

1 Preheat oven to 200°C/180°C fan forced. Line a large baking dish or tray with baking paper. Place the ground coriander, turmeric, mustard seeds and chilli in a bowl and stir to combine. Place potato in the prepared dish and lightly spray with oil. Sprinkle with the turmeric mixture and toss to combine. Bake for 30 minutes.

2 Add the peas, broccolini, capsicums and tomatoes. Stir to combine. Top with the salmon. Bake for 10-12 minutes or until the salmon is cooked to your liking.

3 Meanwhile, combine the yoghurt, lime juice and chopped coriander. Season.

4 Top the tray bake with coriander yoghurt, extra coriander sprigs and lime wedges to serve.

COOK'S NOTE

Not a fan of coriander? Try swapping with fresh mint instead.

NUTRITION (PER SERVE)

CALS	FAT	SAT FAT	PROTEIN	CARBS
420	4g	13.6g	35.5g	22g

★★★★★ *Easy, healthy, tasty meal!* **KYLIE7**

○ VEGETARIAN ○ VEGAN ● GLUTEN FREE ○ MAKE AHEAD ○ FREEZABLE

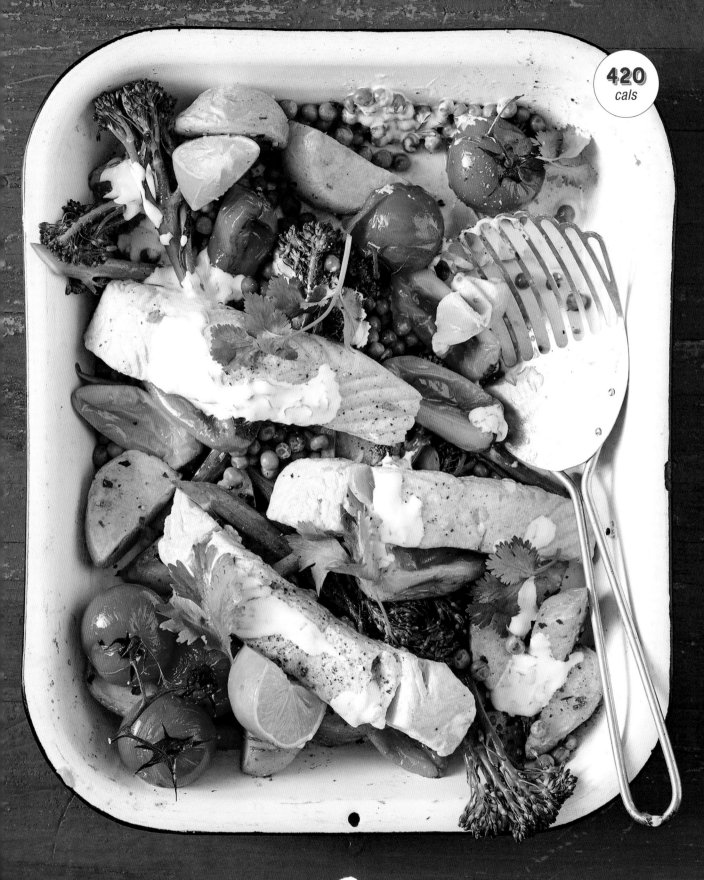

CUMIN-SPICED LAMB &

EGGPLANT

The Mediterranean flavours of this aromatic meat dish
make it perfect for a family meal, or even for entertaining.

SERVES 4 **PREP** 20 mins **COOK** 40 mins

180g (1 cup) freekeh
3 tsp ground cumin
2½ tbs extra virgin olive oil
80ml (⅓ cup) lemon juice
2 small eggplants
280g lamb backstrap
1 small red onion, finely chopped
200g tomato medley mix, halved
⅓ cup fresh mint leaves
¼ cup fresh continental
    parsley leaves
2 tbs fresh dill sprigs
200g tub onion and chive
    cottage cheese

1 Place freekeh and 625ml (2½ cups) water in a medium saucepan over high heat. Bring to the boil. Reduce heat to low. Simmer, covered, for 35-40 minutes or until tender and liquid has been absorbed.

2 Meanwhile, combine cumin, 2 tbs oil and 2 tbs lemon juice in a glass or ceramic dish. Season. Cut eggplant lengthways into 5mm slices. Add eggplant to dish. Rub to coat in spice mixture.

3 Heat a barbecue grill on medium-high heat. Cook eggplant for 3 minutes each side or until charred and tender. Transfer to a large bowl. Add lamb to dish with remaining spice mixture. Toss to coat. Add lamb to grill. Cook for 5 minutes each side for medium, or until cooked to your liking. Transfer to a plate. Cover. Rest lamb for 5 minutes. Slice. Add to eggplant.

4 Add freekeh, red onion, tomato, mint, parsley, dill and remaining lemon juice to bowl with lamb. Season and toss to combine.

5 Spread cottage cheese on serving plate. Top with lamb and eggplant mixture. Drizzle with remaining oil. Serve.

NUTRITION (PER SERVE)

CALS	FAT	SAT FAT	PROTEIN	CARBS
472	15.6g	3.3g	28.2g	46.8g

○ VEGETARIAN   ○ VEGAN   ○ GLUTEN FREE   ○ MAKE AHEAD   ○ FREEZABLE

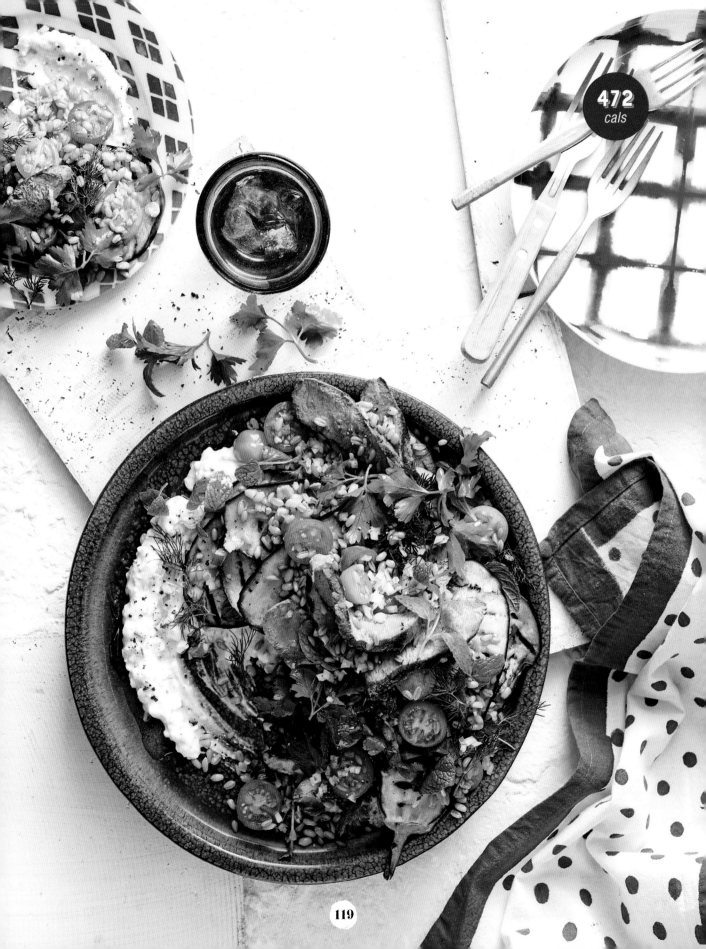

472
cals

LIME & POTATO CURRY WITH FISH

This creamy fish curry is loaded with potato, sweet potato, eggplant and zucchini and has a delicious coconut flavour.

SERVES 4 **PREP** 10 mins **COOKING** 35 mins

450g sweet potato, peeled, cut into 2cm pieces
350g kipfler potatoes, peeled, cut into 2cm pieces
1 large onion, chopped
2 garlic cloves, crushed
1 tbs finely grated fresh ginger
3 tsp finely grated fresh turmeric
275ml gluten-free vegetable stock
250ml (1 cup) light coconut milk
2 Lebanese eggplants, sliced into rounds
2 zucchini, sliced into rounds
600g thick white fish (such as ling), cut into 3cm pieces
1 lime, rind finely grated, juiced, plus extra wedges, to serve
2 tsp fish sauce
Fresh Thai basil leaves, to serve

1 Spray a large non-stick frying pan with oil. Place over medium-high heat. Add sweet potato, potato and onion. Cook, stirring, for 1-2 minutes. Add the garlic, ginger and turmeric. Season well and stir to coat.

2 Add stock and coconut milk. Bring almost to the boil. Reduce heat. Simmer, covered, for 10 minutes. Uncover and simmer for 5 minutes.

3 Add eggplant and zucchini. Simmer, covered, for 10 minutes or until eggplant is tender. Add fish, lime rind, juice and fish sauce. Simmer, covered, for 5 minutes or until fish is cooked through.

4 Divide curry among serving bowls. Top with basil. Serve with extra lime wedges.

NON-FAST DAYS

Add ½ cup steamed brown rice per person. 138 cals per serve.

NUTRITION (PER SERVE)

CALS	FAT	SAT FAT	PROTEIN	CARBS
376	8g	4.5g	35g	34g

○ VEGETARIAN ○ VEGAN ● GLUTEN FREE ● MAKE AHEAD ○ FREEZABLE

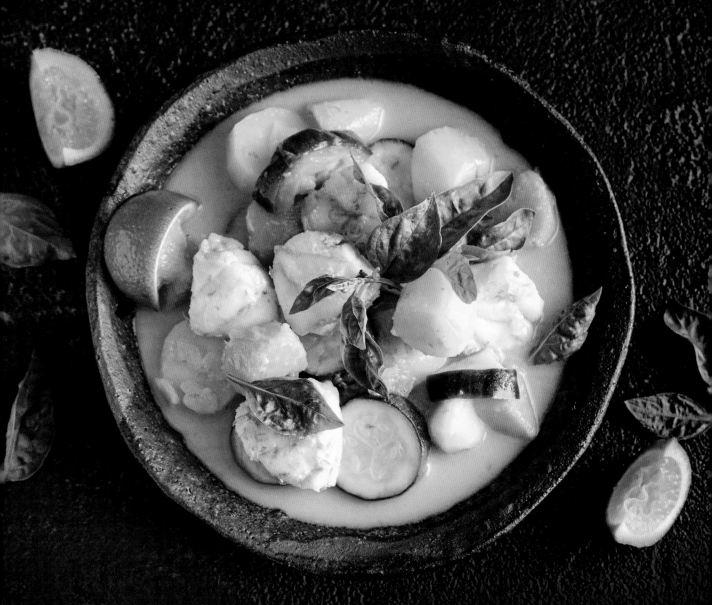

376 cals

★★★★★
This is so easy to make and tastes absolutely delicious!
Even my 6yr old daughter loves it and asks for more! CHEEKYWUN

PUMPKIN FELAFEL WITH SALAD

These delicious and simple pumpkin and chickpea patties are paired with a salad of herbs, tomato and cucumber for added freshness.

SERVES 4 **PREP** 20 mins **COOK** 10 mins

200g peeled pumpkin, steamed, mashed
2 x 400g cans no-added-salt chickpeas, rinsed, drained
1½ tsp ground cumin
1 tsp ground coriander
1 garlic clove, crushed
2 tbs plain flour, plus 1 tbs extra, to dust
½ cup fresh continental parsley leaves, chopped
½ cup fresh mint leaves, chopped
250g cherry tomatoes, chopped
2 Lebanese cucumbers, chopped
2 tsp lemon juice
1 tsp extra virgin olive oil
2 wholemeal pita breads, halved, grilled, to serve
1 lemon, cut into wedges, to serve

1 Place the pumpkin, chickpeas, cumin, coriander, garlic, flour and half the parsley and mint in a food processor and process until finely chopped. Season. Shape the mixture into 24 oval patties. Place the extra flour on a plate. Dust the felafel patties lightly in the flour, shaking off any excess.

2 Place the tomato, cucumber and the remaining parsley and mint in a bowl. Add the lemon juice and olive oil and stir to combine.

3 Spray a large non-stick frying pan with oil and heat over medium-high heat. Cook the felafel for 2-3 minutes each side or until golden brown. Serve the felafel with the salad, grilled bread and lemon wedges.

NON-FAST DAYS

Add 1 medium avocado, sliced, to the salad. 55 cals per serve.

NUTRITION (PER SERVE)

CALS	FAT	SAT FAT	PROTEIN	CARBS
336	6g	1g	14g	50g

● VEGETARIAN ● VEGAN ○ GLUTEN FREE ● MAKE AHEAD ○ FREEZABLE

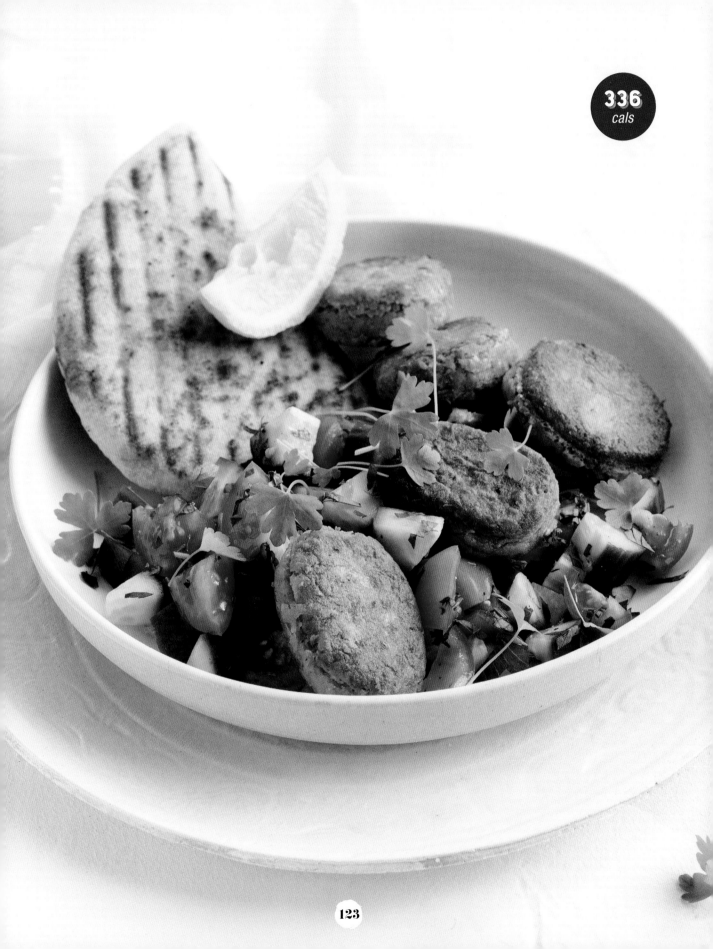

336
cals

123

LIGHT MEALS

TAKE YOUR PICK OF THESE RECIPES.
THEY'RE ALL AROUND 250 CALORIES.

JAPANESE-STYLE CHICKEN SALAD

White miso adds a mild, sweet tang to this speedy shredded chicken and cabbage salad.

SERVES 4 **PREP** 20 mins

400g smoked chicken breast, skin removed, shredded

160g (2 cups) shredded wombok (Chinese cabbage)

1 bunch radishes, trimmed, thinly sliced

2 small zucchini, thinly sliced

1 red apple, unpeeled, cut into matchsticks

¼ small red cabbage, shredded

2 sheets nori, torn

3 tsp white miso paste

1½ tbs mirin

1½ tsp salt-reduced soy sauce

2 tsp sesame oil

Toasted white and black sesame seeds, to serve

1 Combine chicken, wombok, radish, zucchini, apple, red cabbage and nori in a bowl.

2 Whisk together miso, mirin, soy and sesame oil in a small bowl. Drizzle over salad and toss well to combine. Divide among bowls and sprinkle with sesame seeds.

NUTRITION (PER SERVE)

CALS	FAT	SAT FAT	PROTEIN	CARBS
240	5g	1g	32g	14g

NON-FAST DAYS

To make this salad more substantial, cook 180g dried soba noodles. Rinse, drain and toss through salad. 160 cals per serve.

★★★★★ *This is one of my favourite salads! You can mix it up and do a different protein and different salad bits 'n' pieces, but that dressing is the bomb!* **JEN SHIELDS**

○ VEGETARIAN   ○ VEGAN   ○ GLUTEN FREE   ○ MAKE AHEAD   ○ FREEZABLE

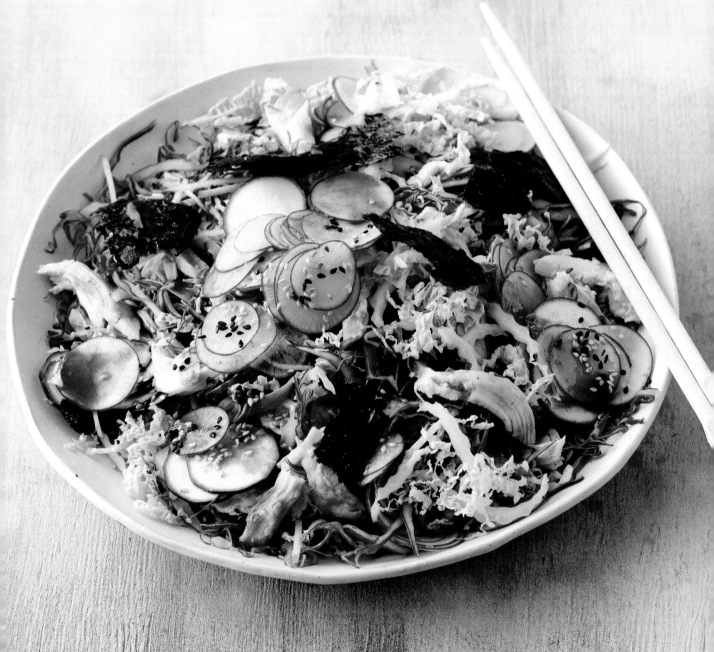

240
cals

SALAD WITH EGG &

RELISH

This easy high-protein, low-cal meal is ideal for brunch, lunch or even a light evening meal.

SERVES 4 **PREP** 10 mins **COOK** 15 mins

3 tsp extra virgin olive oil
1 garlic clove, crushed
1 fresh long red chilli, deseeded, finely chopped
1½ tsp ground cumin
400g can crushed tomatoes
1 tsp maple syrup
8 eggs
2 bunches broccolini, trimmed, cut into 4cm lengths
1 bunch asparagus, trimmed, cut into 4cm lengths
100g mixed salad leaves
2 tsp balsamic vinegar

1 To make the relish, heat 1 tsp oil in a saucepan over medium heat. Cook garlic, chilli and cumin, stirring, for 1 minute. Add tomato and maple syrup. Simmer for 5-10 minutes or until thickened. Season. Set aside to cool.

2 Place eggs in a saucepan. Cover with cold water. Bring to the boil. Reduce heat to low. Simmer for 4 minutes for soft boiled eggs. Drain and refresh under cold running water. Carefully peel eggs and cut in half.

3 Cook broccolini and asparagus in a steamer basket set over a saucepan of boiling water for 4-5 minutes or until tender but crisp. Refresh under cold running water. Drain.

4 Place broccolini, asparagus and salad leaves in a bowl. Drizzle with vinegar and remaining oil. Toss to combine. Divide salad and eggs among plates. Top with tomato relish.

NON-FAST DAYS

Add a 400g can chickpeas, rinsed and drained, to the salad. 68 cals per serve.

NUTRITION (PER SERVE)

CALS	FAT	SAT FAT	PROTEIN	CARBS
233	13g	4g	20g	6g

● VEGETARIAN ○ VEGAN ● GLUTEN FREE ○ MAKE AHEAD ○ FREEZABLE

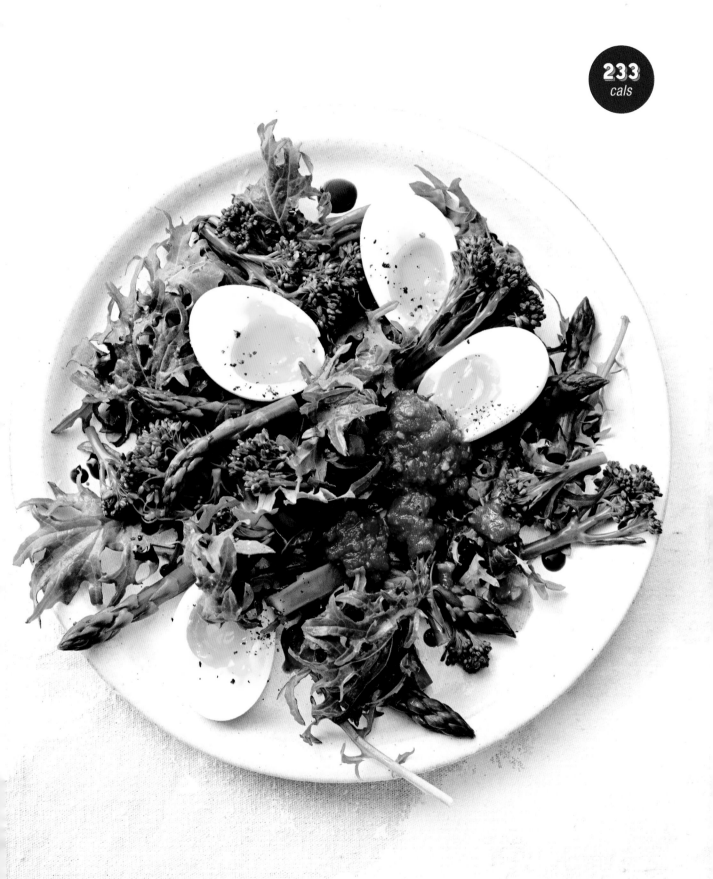

233
cals

129

SPICY KOREAN
PORK

This spicy bowl is packed full of vegies and served on a base of cauliflower rice for more low-carb goodness.

SERVES 4 **PREP** 20 mins (+ 20 mins marinating) **COOK** 20 mins

2 tsp gluten-free gochujang paste
1 tbs gluten-free tamari, plus extra, to serve
2 tsp mirin
1 garlic clove, crushed
500g lean pork fillet, fat trimmed
2 tbs rice wine vinegar
1 tsp caster sugar
1 carrot, cut into noodles using a spiraliser
1 red capsicum, deseeded, thinly sliced
4 large radishes, thinly sliced
1 cucumber, cut into noodles using a spiraliser
1 small head cauliflower, broken into florets
2 tsp sesame oil
80g baby spinach, to serve
Lime cheeks, to serve
Micro herbs and toasted sesame seeds, to serve

1 Combine gochujang paste, tamari, mirin and garlic in a shallow dish. Add pork and turn to coat. Cover and set aside for 20 minutes.

2 Preheat oven to 180°C/160°C fan forced. Line a baking tray. Place a wire rack in tray. Heat a large frying pan over high heat. Cook pork for 1-2 minutes each side, until browned. Place on rack. Brush with remaining marinade. Roast for 12-15 minutes or until cooked to your liking. Transfer to a plate. Cover.

3 Combine rice wine vinegar, sugar and a pinch of salt in a bowl. Add the carrot, capsicum, radish and cucumber. Set aside for 5 minutes.

4 Process the cauliflower in a food processor until mixture resembles rice. Microwave until just tender. Drain. Toss with sesame oil.

5 Serve sliced pork with cauliflower rice, drained carrot mixture, spinach and lime cheeks. Sprinkle with sesame seeds and scatter herbs over. Drizzle with extra tamari.

NON-FAST DAYS

Add 1 medium avocado, sliced, to the salad. 55 cals per serve.

NUTRITION (PER SERVE)

CALS	FAT	SAT FAT	PROTEIN	CARBS
261	6g	1g	34g	13g

○ VEGETARIAN ○ VEGAN ● GLUTEN FREE ○ MAKE AHEAD ○ FREEZABLE

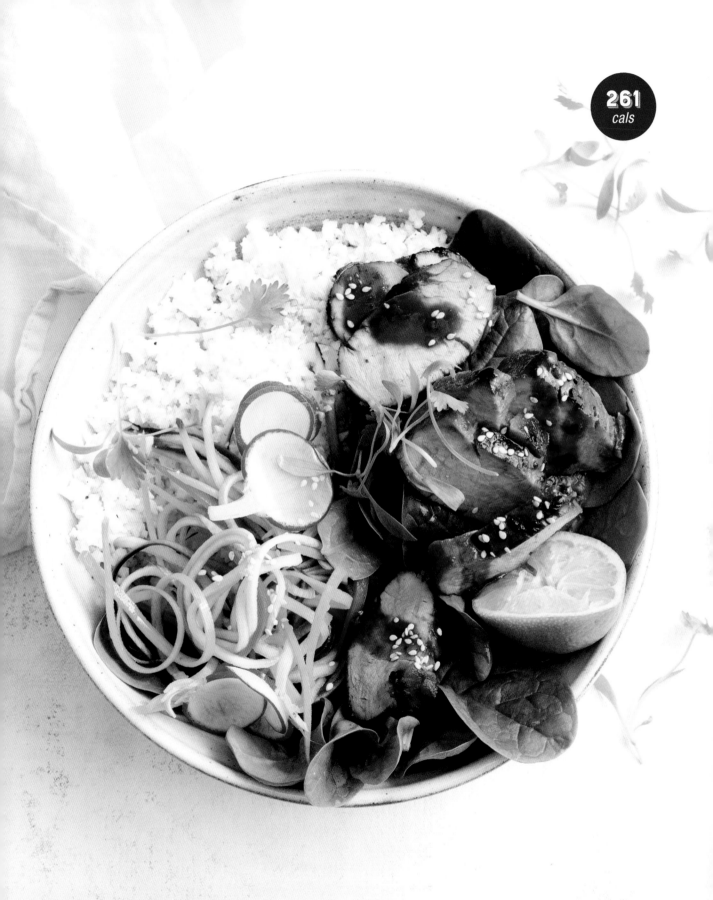

CHICKEN & ZUCCHINI 'LINGUINE'

This better-for-you vegie-packed 'pasta' is actually gluten free and can be ready in just 20 minutes.

SERVES 4 **PREP** 10 mins **COOK** 10 mins

450g chicken breast fillets, halved horizontally
1 tbs olive oil
2 garlic cloves, crushed
500g zucchini noodles
125ml (½ cup) light cream
80ml (⅓ cup) gluten-free chicken stock
1 tbs fresh dill leaves
2 tbs chopped fresh chives
30g baby spinach, to serve
30g parmesan, finely grated

1 Spray a large non-stick frying pan with oil and heat over medium-high heat. Season the chicken well and cook for 2-3 minutes each side or until golden and cooked through. Remove from the pan and keep warm.

2 Heat oil in the pan. Add the garlic and cook, stirring, for 30 seconds. Add the zucchini noodles and cook, stirring, for 1-2 minutes. Add the light cream and chicken stock. Simmer for 1-2 minutes or until the zucchini noodles are just tender but not soft.

3 Slice the chicken and toss through the sauce along with the dill and chives. Divide among serving bowls. Sprinkle with the spinach and parmesan, to serve.

NON-FAST DAYS

Cook 200g dried gluten-free pasta and toss through the sauce. 181 cals per serve.

NUTRITION (PER SERVE)

CALS	FAT	SAT FAT	PROTEIN	CARBS
276	15g	6.5g	29.5g	4g

○ VEGETARIAN ○ VEGAN ● GLUTEN FREE ○ MAKE AHEAD ○ FREEZABLE

★★★★★ *This was so delicious, the sauce is so delicate, but full of flavour. I kept some of the chicken and sauce from the dish and chucked it in a salad the next day – amazing.* **OONALLEE**

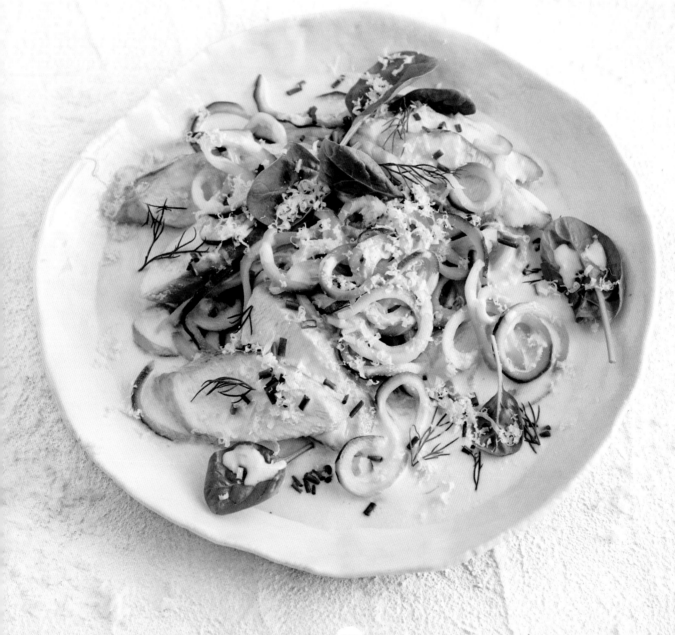

VEGIE & GOAT'S CHEESE
FRITTATA

Use the pick of the season's vegies along with seeds
for added crunch to create this healthy vegetarian meal.

SERVES 6 **PREP** 15 mins (+ cooling) **COOK** 1 hour 15 mins

500g butternut pumpkin, peeled,
   deseeded, cut into 1.5cm pieces
1 large red capsicum, deseeded,
   cut into 1.5cm pieces
1 large red onion, cut into thin wedges
1 bunch asparagus, trimmed,
   cut into 1cm lengths
150g (1 cup) frozen green peas
75g soft goat's cheese, crumbled
8 eggs
2 tbs milk
¼ cup chopped fresh basil leaves,
   plus extra baby leaves, to serve
150g mixed cherry tomatoes, halved
1 tbs sunflower and pumpkin seeds

1 Preheat oven to 200°C/180°C fan forced. Line a large baking tray with baking paper. Place pumpkin, capsicum and onion on prepared tray. Spray lightly with olive oil. Roast for 25-30 minutes or until golden and tender. Set aside to cool.

2 Meanwhile, place asparagus and peas in a steamer basket over a saucepan of boiling water. Cover and steam until tender crisp. Refresh vegetables under cold running water. Drain well.

3 Reserve 1 tbs goat's cheese. Place remaining goat's cheese in a large bowl with eggs, milk and basil. Whisk to combine. Season. Add all of the cooked vegetables and stir to combine.

4 Reduce oven to 180°C/160°C fan forced. Line base and side of 20cm round cake pan with baking paper. Pour mixture into prepared pan, evenly distributing veg. Top with tomato, cut-side up, and seeds. Bake for 45 minutes or until puffed and firm. Set aside for 10 minutes to cool. Top with extra basil and reserved cheese. Serve with salad, if you like.

NUTRITION (PER SERVE)

CALS	FAT	SAT FAT	PROTEIN	CARBS
225	11g	3.5g	17g	12g

● VEGETARIAN ○ VEGAN ● GLUTEN FREE ○ MAKE AHEAD ○ FREEZABLE

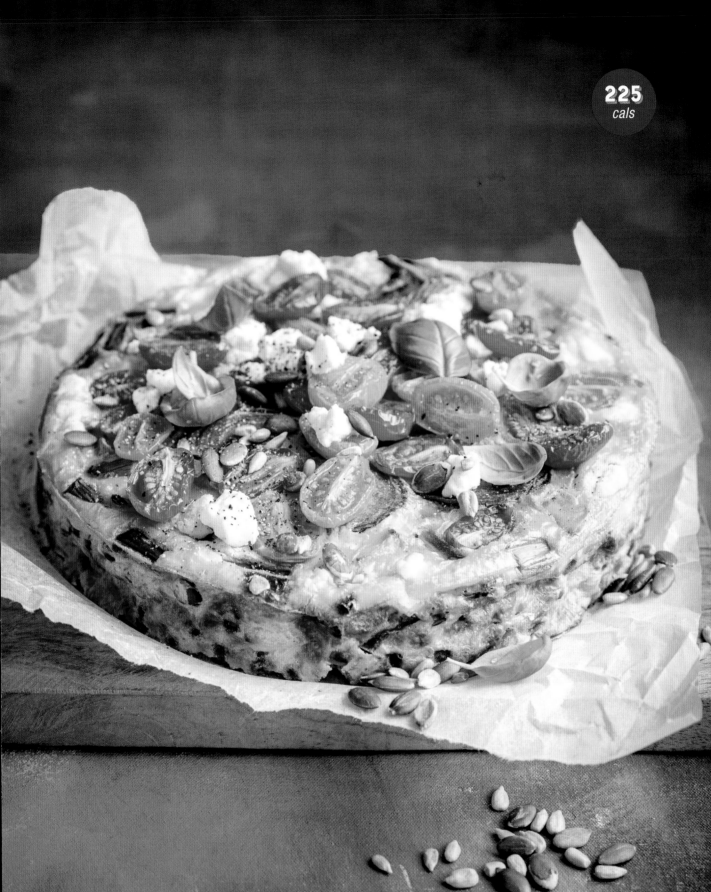

KALE WITH EGG & SWEET POTATO

This good-for-you, fast and hearty breakfast combo will get the tastebuds firing – and rival the menu of any café.

SERVES 2 **PREP** 5 mins **COOK** 25 mins

300g peeled sweet potato, cut
  crossways into 1cm slices
1 tsp extra virgin olive oil
1 garlic clove, thinly sliced
75g trimmed kale, coarsely chopped
2 eggs, poached
1 tbs natural almonds, sliced

1 Preheat oven to 200°C/180°C fan forced. Line a baking tray with baking paper. Place potato on prepared tray. Lightly spray with olive oil. Roast for 20-25 minutes or until golden and tender.

2 Meanwhile, heat oil in a large non-stick frying pan over medium-high heat. Cook garlic, stirring, for 30 seconds or until aromatic. Add kale and stir until just wilted.

3 Divide the sweet potato among serving plates. Top with the wilted kale mixture and poached eggs. Sprinkle with the almonds. Serve.

NON-FAST DAYS

Toss 1 cup rinsed and drained chickpeas in with the garlic and kale. 98 cals per serve.

NUTRITION (PER SERVE)

CALS	FAT	SAT FAT	PROTEIN	CARBS
256	12g	2g	11g	23g

● VEGETARIAN ○ VEGAN ● GLUTEN FREE ○ MAKE AHEAD ○ FREEZABLE

256
cals

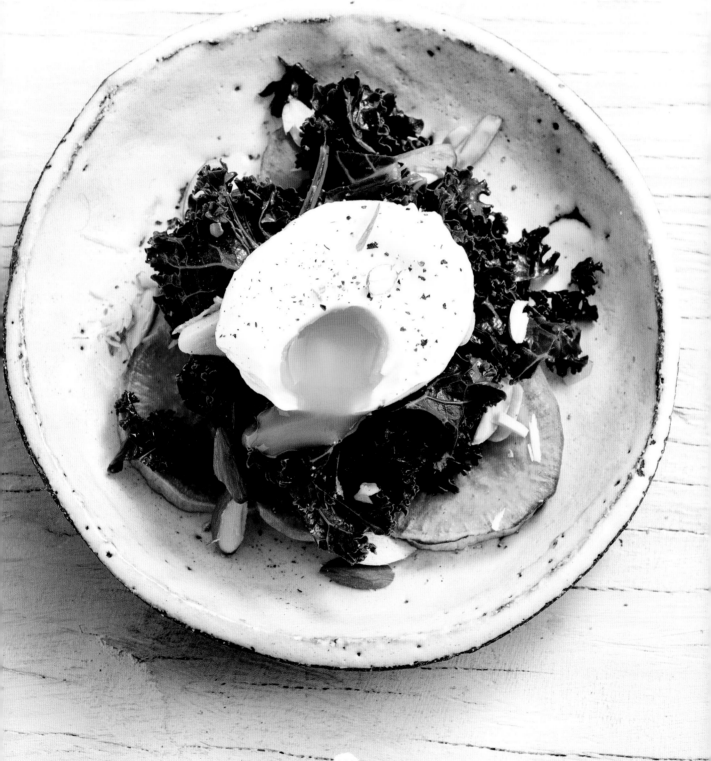

WHITE BEAN PANCAKES & BERRIES

The inclusion of cannellini beans in these pancakes gives them a healthy and filling twist. Top with your favourite fruits for a fresh surprise.

SERVES 4 **PREP** 15 mins (+ 10 mins standing) **COOK** 20 mins

400g can cannellini beans, rinsed, drained
2 eggs
2 tbs maple syrup
½ tsp vanilla extract
150g (1 cup) wholemeal self-raising flour
185ml (¾ cup) reduced-fat milk
1 tsp melted butter, to brush
150g strawberries, quartered
Pulp of 2 passionfruit

1 Process beans until smooth. Add eggs, 1 tbs maple syrup and vanilla. Process until well combined. Transfer to a bowl. Sift over flour. Return husks to bowl. Add milk and whisk until smooth. Set aside for 10 minutes.

2 Heat a large non-stick frying pan over medium-high heat. Brush lightly with butter. Ladle two quarter-cupfuls of batter into pan. Cook for 3 minutes or until bubbles appear. Turn and cook for 1 minute until light golden. Transfer to a plate and keep warm. Repeat to make 8 pancakes. Top with strawberries, passionfruit pulp and remaining maple syrup.

NON-FAST DAYS

Top with 1½ tbs natural yoghurt per person.
25 cals per serve.

NUTRITION (PER SERVE)

CALS	FAT	SAT FAT	PROTEIN	CARBS
298	5g	2g	13g	44g

★★★★★ *Made this recipe a few times now and cannot tell the base is cannellini beans. I know it's healthier and with a drizzle of passionfruit it adds a slight tartness. Delish! Kids couldn't tell and ate the lot.* **FOODIEPLUS**

● VEGETARIAN ○ VEGAN ○ GLUTEN FREE ○ MAKE AHEAD ○ FREEZABLE

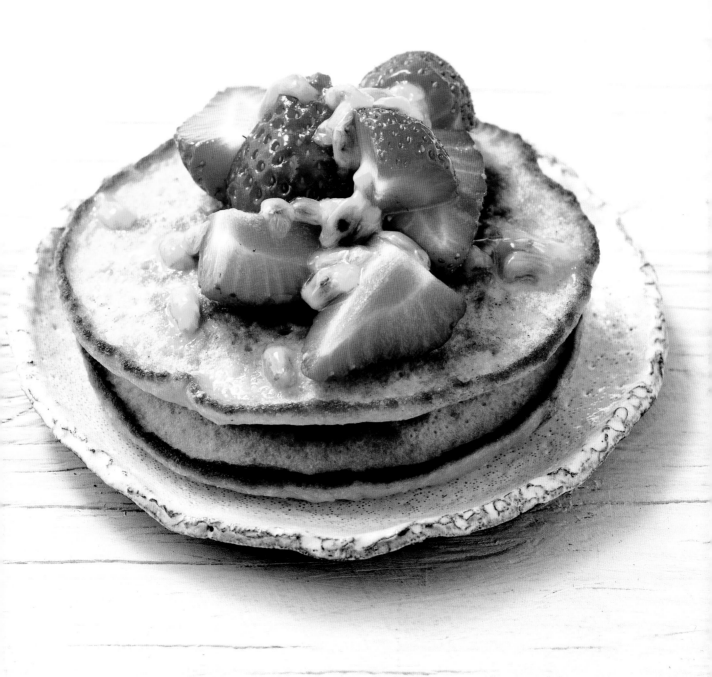

298
cals

BARLEY, GINGER & MISO SOUP

This slow-cooked barley soup contains ginger as well as miso paste for a delicious umami flavour. Even better, there's minimal prep required.

SERVES 4 **PREP** 15 mins **COOK** 1 hour

2 tsp macadamia oil
1 large onion, finely chopped
3 celery sticks, trimmed, diced
2 carrots, peeled, diced
1 tbs finely grated fresh ginger
3 garlic cloves, thinly sliced
110g (½ cup) pearl barley, rinsed, drained
1½ tbs miso paste
400g frozen edamame, thawed, podded
1 bunch broccolini, trimmed, cut into 3cm lengths
1 tsp tamari
Chopped fresh chives, to serve

1 Heat the oil in a large saucepan over medium heat. Cook the onion, celery and carrot, stirring often, for 6-7 minutes or until softened. Add the ginger and garlic and cook, stirring, for 1 minute or until aromatic. Add the barley and stir to combine.

2 Add the miso paste and 1.25L (5 cups) water and bring to the boil. Reduce the heat to low, cover and simmer for 45 minutes.

3 Add edamame and broccolini. Simmer, uncovered, for 5 minutes or until the vegetables are just tender. Stir through the tamari and season. Sprinkle with chives to serve.

NON-FAST DAYS

Serve with 1 slice wholegrain sourdough bread per person 91 cals per serve.

NUTRITION (PER SERVE)

CALS	FAT	SAT FAT	PROTEIN	CARBS
196	4g	1g	6g	27g

○ VEGETARIAN ● **VEGAN** ○ GLUTEN FREE ○ MAKE AHEAD ○ FREEZABLE

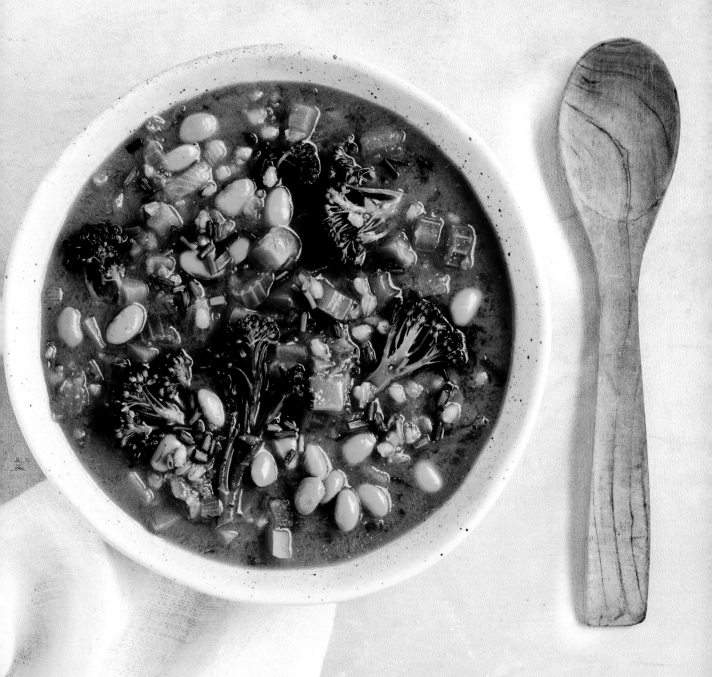

196
cals

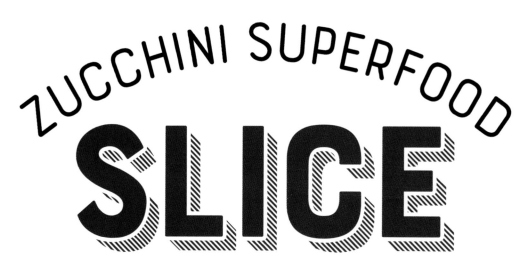

ZUCCHINI SUPERFOOD SLICE

This healthy version of zucchini slice is loaded with quinoa, zucchini and kale, and makes a perfect dinner or lunchbox filler.

SERVES 6 **PREP** 20 mins **COOK** 30 mins

2 tsp olive oil
1 brown onion, finely chopped
2 garlic cloves, crushed
2 carrots, trimmed, coarsely grated
150g chopped kale
8 eggs
85g (⅓ cup) reduced-fat
   ricotta cheese
3 zucchini, finely grated, squeezed
   of excess moisture
2 tbs chopped fresh
   continental parsley
150g (1 cup) cooked quinoa
200g grape tomatoes, halved

1 Preheat oven to 180/160C fan-forced. Lightly spray a 20 x 30cm baking pan with oil and line the base with baking paper, allowing the 2 long sides to overhang.

2 Heat the oil in a large non-stick frying pan over medium heat. Add the onion and cook, stirring often, for 3-4 minutes or until softened. Add the garlic and carrot and cook, stirring, for 1 minute or until garlic is aromatic. Add the kale and cook, stirring, for 3 minutes or until wilted. Season and set aside for 5 minutes to cool slightly.

3 Whisk the eggs and ricotta together in a large bowl. Add the cooled vegetables, zucchini, parsley and quinoa. Season. Spoon the mixture into the prepared pan. Top with tomatoes, cut side up. Bake for 25-30 minutes or until golden and puffed and firm to the touch. Set aside for 10 minutes to cool, before cutting into 6 slices to serve.

NUTRITION (PER SERVE)

CALS	FAT	SAT FAT	PROTEIN	CARBS
192	9.4g	2.9g	12.9g	9.8g

○ VEGETARIAN   ○ VEGAN   ● GLUTEN FREE   ● MAKE AHEAD   ○ FREEZABLE

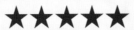

★★★★★

We really enjoyed this slice – easy to make and very satisfying. **DEBFRENCH**

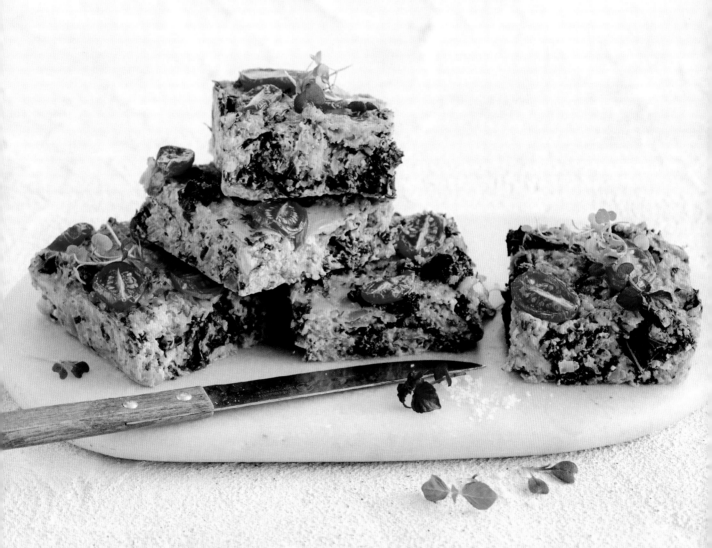

ROSEMARY & LEMON
STEAK

Easy and using classic flavour combos, this steak dish is perfect as a midweek meal and the white bean salad is a healthy alternative to chips.

SERVES 4 **PREP** 10 mins (+ 30 mins marinating) **COOK** 10 mins

2 tsp finely chopped fresh rosemary
1½ tsp finely grated lemon rind
1½ tbs fresh lemon juice
1 tbs extra virgin olive oil
2 x 250g lean sirloin steaks,
   fat trimmed
350g tomato medley mix
2 bunches asparagus, trimmed
400g can cannellini beans,
   rinsed, drained

1 Combine rosemary, 1 tsp rind, 1 tbs lemon juice and 2 tsp oil in a glass or ceramic dish. Add steaks and turn to coat. Cover and set aside for 30 minutes to marinate.

2 Preheat barbecue grill or chargrill pan on medium-high. Brush steaks with 1 tsp oil. Cook for 2-3 minutes each side for medium or until cooked to your liking. Set aside, covered loosely, for 4 minutes to rest. Slice.

3 Meanwhile, lightly spray the tomatoes and asparagus with olive oil. Cook for 1-2 minutes each side or until tender. Combine tomatoes, beans and remaining rind, lemon juice and oil in a bowl. Season.

4 Serve the steaks over a bed of asparagus and the white bean salad.

NON-FAST DAYS

Serve with 1 slice gluten-free multigrain bread per person.
93 cals per serve.

NUTRITION (PER SERVE)

CALS	FAT	SAT FAT	PROTEIN	CARBS
270	9g	2g	33g	10g

○ VEGETARIAN   ○ VEGAN   ● GLUTEN FREE   ○ MAKE AHEAD   ○ FREEZABLE

270 *cals*

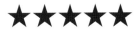
★ ★ ★ ★ ★

This is one of our favourite steak dishes – simple, but the marinade gives the steak a lovely fresh lemon and rosemary flavour. **BONDAS**

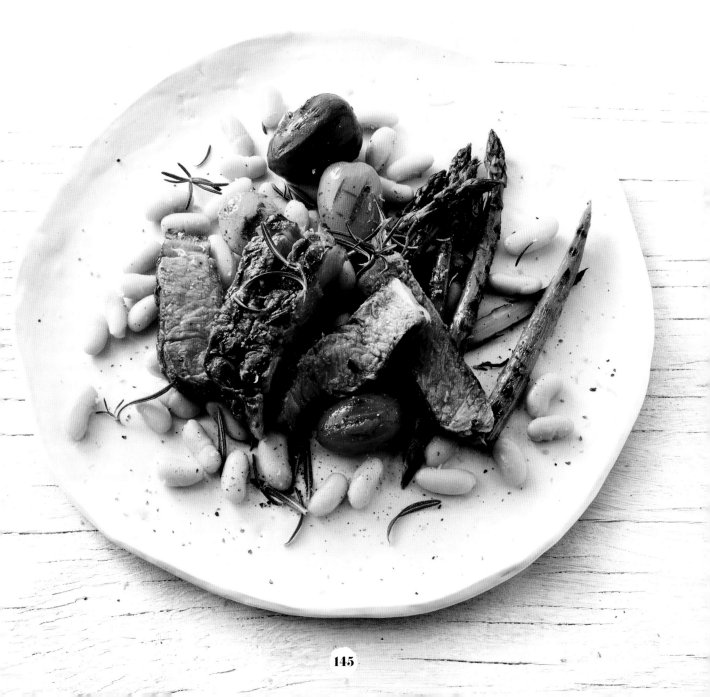

SOUP WITH LEMON &

TURMERIC

This vegetarian soup gets its lovely golden colour from turmeric, which contains curcumin, known for its anti-inflammatory properties.

SERVES 4 **PREP** 15 mins **COOK** 45 mins

2 tsp extra virgin olive oil
1 large red onion, finely chopped
3 celery sticks, finely chopped
2 garlic cloves, crushed
2 tsp finely grated lemon rind
1 tsp ground turmeric
½ tsp ground cinnamon
½ tsp dried chilli flakes
500ml (2 cups) gluten-free
    salt-reduced vegetable stock
135g (¾ cup) French green lentils,
    rinsed, drained
2 vine-ripened tomatoes, chopped
150g green beans, trimmed, sliced
100g trimmed kale, chopped
1 tbs fresh lemon juice
2 tbs chopped fresh coriander

1 Heat the olive oil in a large saucepan over medium heat. Add the onion and celery. Cook, stirring occasionally, for 5 minutes or until softened. Add the garlic, lemon rind, turmeric, cinnamon and chilli flakes. Cook, stirring, for 1 minute or until aromatic.

2 Add stock, lentils, tomato and 750ml (3 cups) water to the pan. Bring to the boil. Reduce the heat to low and partially cover. Simmer for 30 minutes, until lentils are tender.

3 Add the beans and kale to the soup. Stir to combine. Simmer for 3-4 minutes or until the beans are tender crisp. Stir in the lemon juice and season with pepper. Stir in the coriander just before serving.

NON-FAST DAYS

Top each bowl with 2 tbs unsweetened coconut yoghurt. 62 cals per serve.

NUTRITION (PER SERVE)

CALS	FAT	SAT FAT	PROTEIN	CARBS
197	4g	1g	12g	24g

● VEGETARIAN ● VEGAN ● GLUTEN FREE ● MAKE AHEAD ● FREEZABLE

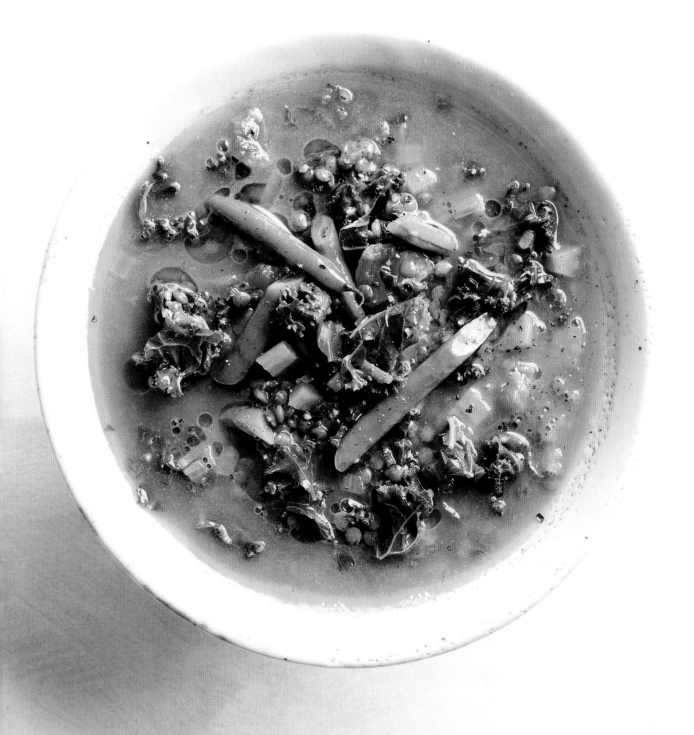

SAVOURY FRENCH TOAST

Who says French toast has to be sweet? This deliciously eggy version pairs brekkie fave avocado with juicy cherry tomatoes.

SERVES 2 **PREP** 10 mins **COOK** 10 mins

125g cherry truss tomatoes
2 eggs
2 tbs milk
4 small (25g each) slices wholemeal sourdough bread
½ small avocado, sliced
¼ cup fresh basil leaves

1 Preheat the oven to 180°C/160°C fan forced. Line a baking tray with baking paper.

2 Place tomatoes on the prepared tray and roast for 10 minutes or until slightly wilted. Whisk together the eggs and milk in a large shallow bowl.

3 Lightly spray a large non-stick frying pan with oil and heat over medium heat. Dip 2 bread slices, 1 at a time, in egg mixture until well soaked. Cook for 2 minutes each side or until golden brown and egg is set. Repeat with remaining bread and egg mixture.

4 Serve the French toast topped with tomatoes, avocado and fresh basil leaves.

NON-FAST DAYS

For added protein and an omega-3 boost, add 2 slices of smoked salmon per person. 94 cals per serve.

NUTRITION (PER SERVE)

CALS	FAT	SAT FAT	PROTEIN	CARBS
253	15g	4g	12g	15g

● **VEGETARIAN** ○ VEGAN ○ GLUTEN FREE ○ MAKE AHEAD ○ FREEZABLE

253
cals

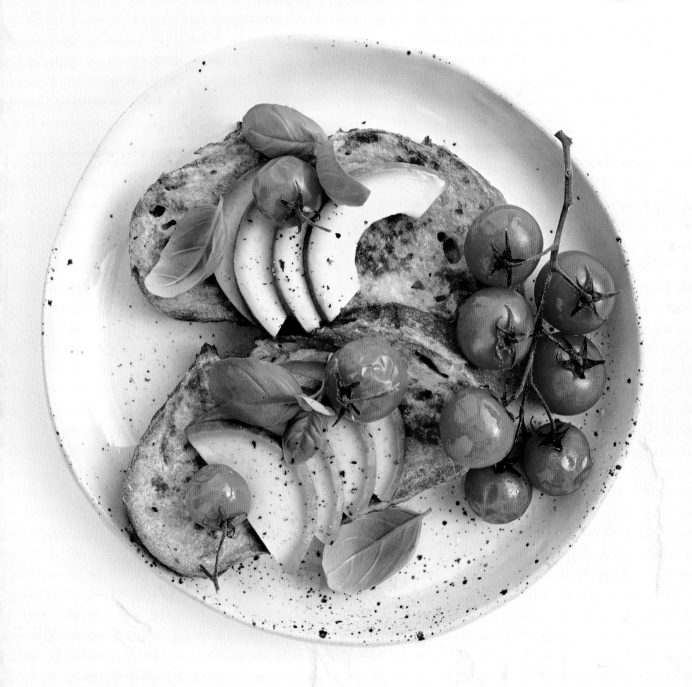

WATERMELON & BERRY
SALAD

With buckwheat and pistachios for crunch, this sugar-free salad has the best of the summer fruits – and is packed with vitamin C.

SERVES 4 **PREP** 10 mins **COOK** 5 mins

2 tbs raw buckwheat kernels
2 tbs shredded coconut
2 tbs pistachios, coarsely chopped
800g seedless watermelon, skin removed, cut into wedges
250g strawberries, hulled, halved
125g fresh raspberries
190g (⅔ cup) natural yoghurt, to serve

1 Preheat the oven to 180°C/160°C fan forced. Line a baking tray with baking paper. Combine the buckwheat, coconut and pistachio in a bowl. Spread the buckwheat mixture over the prepared tray and bake, stirring once, for 5 minutes or until light golden.

2 Arrange the watermelon, strawberry and raspberries on serving plates. Sprinkle each with a little of the buckwheat mixture and top with a dollop of yoghurt.

NON-FAST DAYS

Double the yoghurt and drizzle each serve with 1 tsp honey. 59 cals per serve.

NUTRITION (PER SERVE)

CALS	FAT	SAT FAT	PROTEIN	CARBS
188	7g	4g	7g	22g

Nutrition tip *We all know berries are superfoods, but don't forget watermelon. It's low in calories, rich in vitamin C and potassium, and contains pectin, a type of soluble fibre that may help maintain healthy blood cholesterol levels.* **CHRISSY FREER**

● VEGETARIAN ○ VEGAN ● GLUTEN FREE ○ MAKE AHEAD ○ FREEZABLE

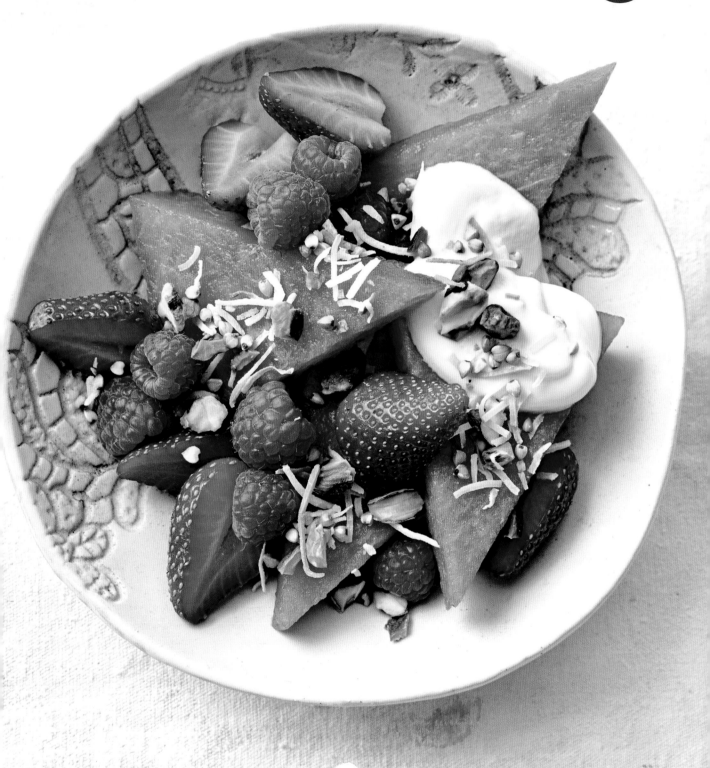

STICKY PORK WITH ZOODLES

Tossed with crisp vegies, zucchini noodles and aromatic herbs, this marinated sweet and sticky pork feels indulgent, while still being good for you.

SERVES 4 **PREP** 15 mins (+15 mins marinating) **COOK** 10 mins

2 tbs kecap manis
1 tbs coconut sugar
1½ tbs fish sauce
500g pork fillet, thinly sliced
1 tbs coconut oil
1 red onion, cut into thin wedges
1 bunch broccolini, halved
4cm piece fresh ginger, peeled,
   cut into matchsticks
2 garlic cloves, thinly sliced
1 lemongrass stem, pale section
   only, finely chopped
1 fresh long red chilli, thinly sliced
200g snow peas, trimmed
500g zucchini, cut into noodles
   using a spiraliser
1 small bunch fresh Thai basil or
   coriander, leaves picked
Lime halves, to serve

1 Combine the kecap manis, sugar and fish sauce in a glass or ceramic bowl. Add pork. Stir to coat. Set aside for 15 minutes (or up to 1 day) to marinate.

2 Drain pork from marinade, reserving marinade. Heat 1 tsp of the oil in a wok over high heat. Add half the pork. Stir-fry for 1-2 minutes or until browned. Transfer pork to a bowl. Repeat with 1 tsp oil and remaining pork.

3 Heat remaining oil in wok over high heat. Add onion and broccolini stems. Stir-fry for 1 minute. Add broccolini florets, ginger, garlic, lemongrass and chilli. Stir-fry for 30 seconds or until aromatic. Add reserved marinade and stir-fry for 1 minute or until vegetables are tender-crisp. Add the snow peas. Stir-fry for 30 seconds. Add zucchini noodles. Stir-fry for 1 minute or until well combined and just tender. Remove from heat.

4 Stir through half the Thai basil. Serve with lime halves and scatter remaining Thai basil over.

NON-FAST DAYS

Serve with ½ cup steamed brown rice per person. 138 cals per serve.

NUTRITION (PER SERVE)

CALS	FAT	SAT FAT	PROTEIN	CARBS
267	7g	5g	36g	12g

○ VEGETARIAN ○ VEGAN ○ GLUTEN FREE ○ MAKE AHEAD ○ FREEZABLE

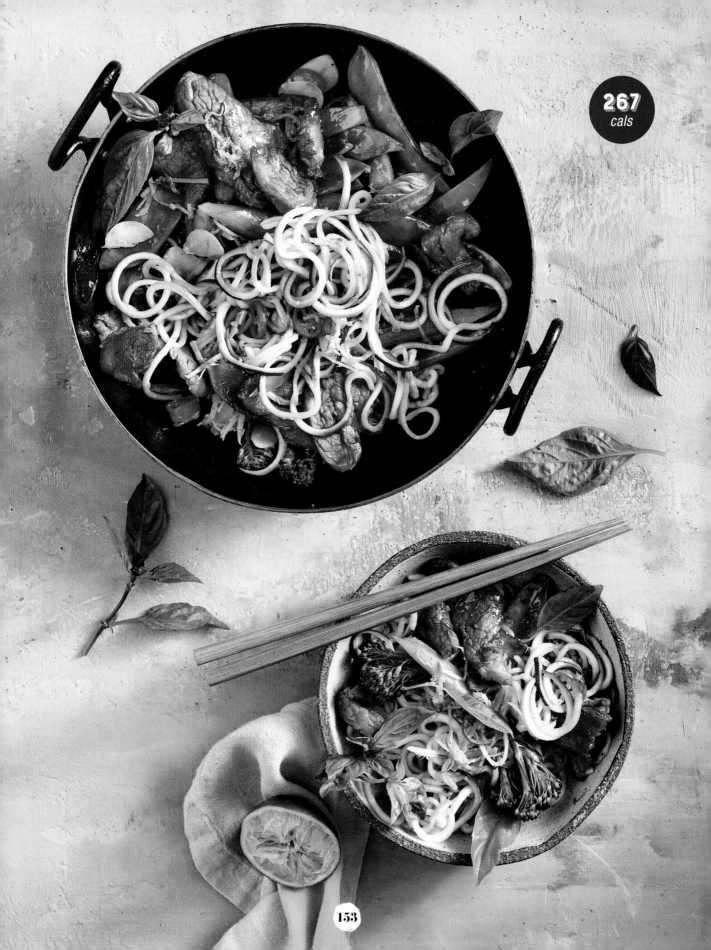

267
cals

EGGPLANT WITH PISTACHIO &
MINT

This deliciously fresh salad includes barbecued eggplant and is gluten-free, vegetarian and low cal.

SERVES 4 **PREP** 15 mins **COOK** 10 mins

2 tbs gluten-free tamari
1 tsp smoked paprika
1 tsp ground coriander
1 lime, rind finely grated, juiced, plus extra lime wedges, to serve
1½ tbs pure maple syrup
150g snow peas, thinly sliced
320g (2 cups) cooked quinoa
2 vine-ripened tomatoes, deseeded, chopped
½ cup fresh mint leaves, chopped, plus extra, to serve
½ cup fresh continental parsley, chopped, plus extra, to serve
2 eggplants, cut crossways into 1.5cm-thick slices
2 tbs pistachios, chopped

1 Combine the tamari, paprika, coriander, lime rind and juice, and 2 tsp maple syrup in a bowl. Set aside.

2 Place the snow peas in a heatproof bowl. Pour in enough boiling water to cover and set aside for 10 seconds. Drain and refresh under cold running water. Drain.

3 Combine the quinoa, snow peas, tomato, mint, parsley and half the marinade in a large bowl. Season.

4 Preheat a barbecue plate or chargrill pan on medium-high. Add the remaining 1 tbs maple syrup to the remaining marinade. Lightly spray the eggplant with oil. Cook, brushing regularly with the marinade, for 4 minutes each side, or until tender and sticky.

5 Arrange eggplant on the quinoa salad. Sprinkle with pistachios and extra herbs and serve with lime wedges.

NON-FAST DAYS

Add 25g crumbled feta or vegan cheese to each serve. 70 cals per serve.

NUTRITION (PER SERVE)

CALS	FAT	SAT FAT	PROTEIN	CARBS
238	6g	1g	10g	30g

● VEGETARIAN ● VEGAN ● GLUTEN FREE ○ MAKE AHEAD ○ FREEZABLE

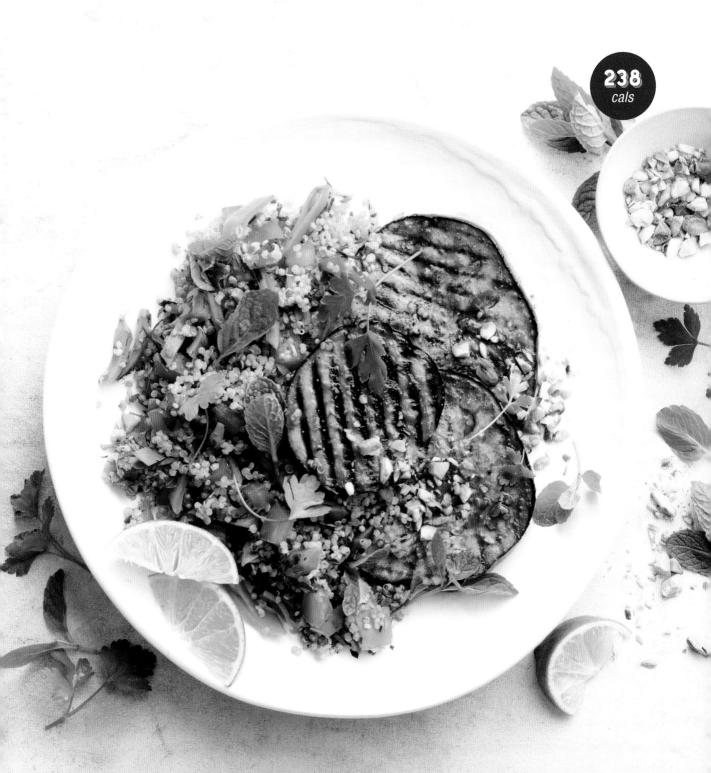

238 cals

★★★★★ *Found it very tasty — I changed the lime rind and juice to a lemon and added more maple syrup.* TRISHA

SOUP WITH CHICKEN & QUINOA

The heat of harissa adds a great kick and Middle Eastern twist to this hearty and satisfying soup.

SERVES 4 **PREP** 15 mins **COOK** 1 hour 35 mins

1.3kg free-range chicken
1 leek, sliced
3 celery sticks, coarsely chopped
10 black peppercorns
4 garlic cloves, peeled
Handful fresh continental
    parsley stalks
70g (⅓ cup) quinoa, rinsed, drained
1 large carrot, peeled,
    finely chopped
1 large zucchini, trimmed,
    finely chopped
75g baby spinach leaves
Harissa (optional), to serve

1 Rinse chicken cavity. Place in a large saucepan with the leek, celery, peppercorns, garlic and parsley. Cover with cold water. Slowly bring to boil over medium heat. Skim fat from surface. Reduce heat to low. Partially cover. Simmer for 1 hour. Remove chicken. Set aside to cool slightly. Simmer stock for a further 15 minutes to develop the flavours.

2 Strain stock through a sieve over a bowl. Discard solids. When chicken is cool enough to handle, remove and discard skin and bones. Shred meat from breasts and thighs, and set aside. Save remaining meat for another meal.

3 Place 1.5L of the stock in a saucepan over high heat. Bring to boil. Reduce heat to medium. Add quinoa. Simmer for 15 minutes or until tender. Add carrot, zucchini and shredded chicken. Simmer for 5 minutes or until vegies are tender. Stir spinach through until it wilts. Season. Stir in a little harissa, if using.

NON-FAST DAYS

Serve with 1 slice gluten-free multigrain bread per person. 93 cals per serve.

NUTRITION (PER SERVE)

CALS	FAT	SAT FAT	PROTEIN	CARBS
253	6g	2g	35g	13g

○ VEGETARIAN ○ VEGAN ● GLUTEN FREE ● MAKE AHEAD ● FREEZABLE

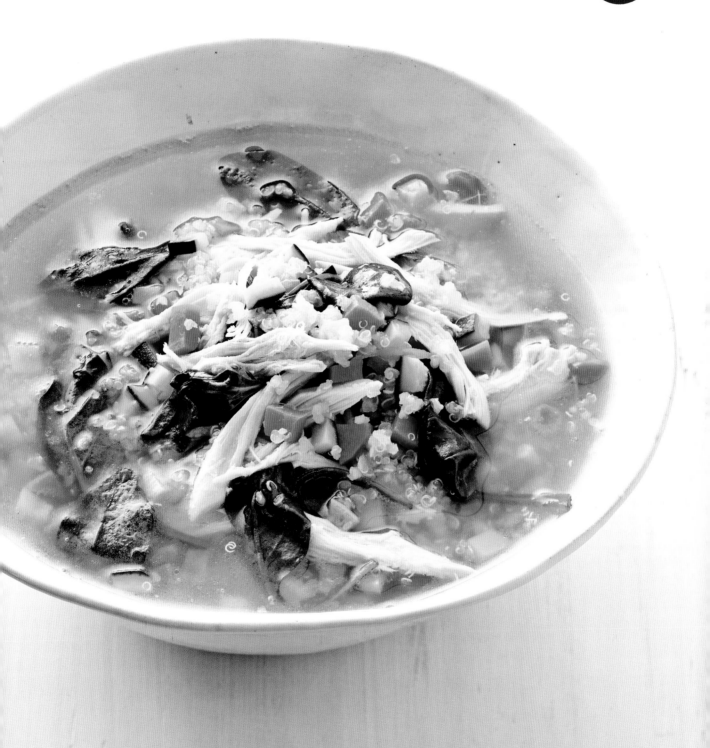

253
cals

BANANA & BLUEBERRY
TOAST

Totally tempting, yet stunningly simple, this topping for sourdough toast will have you out the door in 10 minutes.

SERVES 1 **PREP** 5 mins **COOK** 5 mins

2 small (25g each) slices wholemeal
    sourdough bread, toasted
2 tsp nut butter
Pinch of ground cinnamon
½ banana, sliced
35g (¼ cup) fresh blueberries

1 Spread toast with nut butter. Sprinkle with cinnamon. Top with banana and blueberries.

NUTRITION (PER SERVE)

CALS	FAT	SAT FAT	PROTEIN	CARBS
267	8g	1g	10g	35g

NON-FAST DAYS

Double the amount of nut butter and drizzle with 1 tsp honey. 88 cals.

★★★★★

This was a great breakfast – we will be having this once a week for sure. **CAMSTAR**

● VEGETARIAN ● VEGAN ○ GLUTEN FREE ○ MAKE AHEAD ○ FREEZABLE

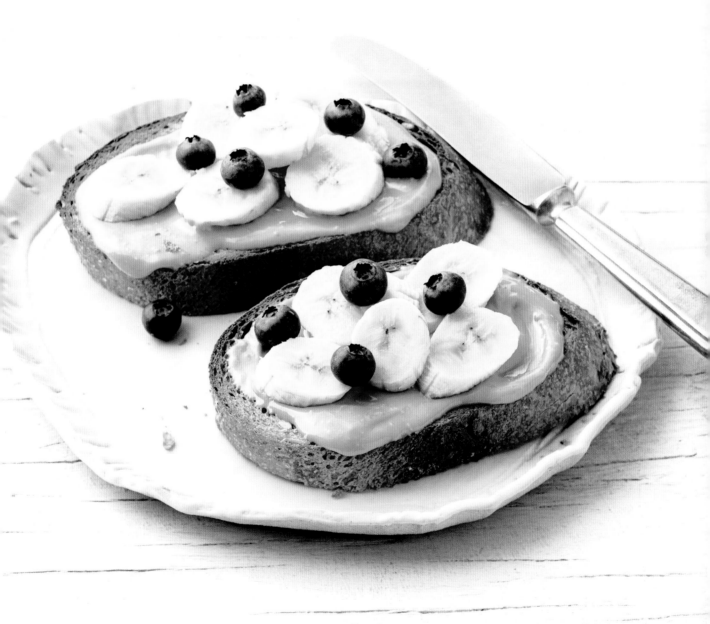

267
cals

159

STICKY BEEF & BEAN
STIR-FRY

Ready in only 20 minutes, this simple stir-fry includes lean mince plus pineapple juice for a sweet hit.

SERVES 4 **PREP** 10 mins **COOK** 20 mins

3 garlic cloves, sliced
500g lean beef mince
2 tbs Thai stir-in seasoning
250ml (1 cup) pineapple juice
1 tbs oyster sauce
2 tsp coconut sugar
350g green beans, trimmed, sliced
1 cup fresh coriander sprigs
⅓ cup chopped fresh mint leaves
2 long fresh red chillies, thinly sliced

1 Heat a large frying pan over medium heat. Spray with oil. Cook garlic for 1-2 minutes, until lightly golden. Transfer to a plate. Set aside. Add beef. Stir-fry for 5 minutes, until browned.

2 Add seasoning. Cook, stirring, for 1 minute. Add pineapple juice, oyster sauce and sugar. Simmer, stirring often, for 10 minutes or until the liquid reduces and the mixture is dark golden and sticky.

3 Add the beans and cook, stirring often, for 1-2 minutes, until tender crisp. Stir through the coriander and mint. Sprinkle with chilli and garlic.

NON-FAST DAYS

Serve with ½ cup steamed brown rice per person. 138 cals per serve.

NUTRITION (PER SERVE)

CALS	FAT	SAT FAT	PROTEIN	CARBS
275	8g	3g	32g	16g

★★★★★ *You know you are onto a winner when there is nothing to keep as leftovers. This is a super simple and tasty dish that will definitely be made again and again.* **LEIANNA**

○ VEGETARIAN ○ VEGAN ○ GLUTEN FREE ○ MAKE AHEAD ○ FREEZABLE

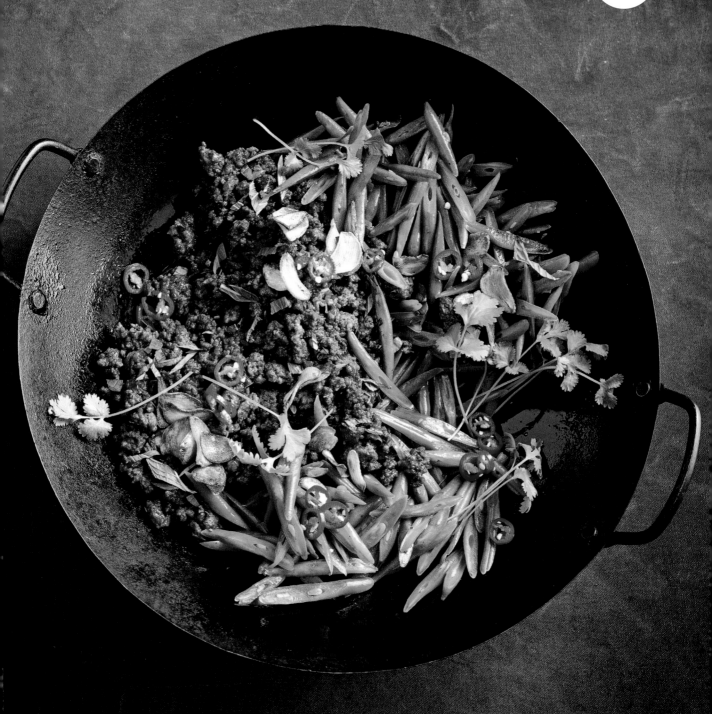

275 cals

PIRI PIRI FISH & CHARRED CORN

Fire up the barbecue and serve up this deliciously healthy fish meal – super simple and ready in only 30 minutes.

SERVES 4   **PREP** 15 mins   **COOK** 15 mins

2 tsp finely grated lime rind
2 tsp smoked paprika
½-1 tsp dried red chilli flakes, to taste
4 x 150g firm white fish fillets
3 sweet corn cobs, husk and silks removed
2 limes, halved
250g cherry tomatoes, halved
150g snow peas, sliced
½ avocado, chopped
2 cups picked watercress sprigs
½ cup fresh coriander leaves
2 tsp fresh lime juice

1 Combine the rind, paprika and chilli flakes in a small bowl. Sprinkle the spice mixture evenly over the fish fillets.

2 Preheat a barbecue grill and flat plate on medium-high. Spray corn, lime halves and fish with olive oil. Cook corn on grill, turning, for 8 minutes or until lightly charred and tender. Cool slightly. Cut kernels from cobs.

3 Combine the tomato, snow pea, avocado, watercress, coriander, corn kernels and lime juice in a large bowl.

4 Cook the fish on the flat plate, turning, for 2-3 minutes each side or until just cooked through. Transfer to a plate. Cook the lime halves on grill, flesh side down, for 1 minute or until charred. Serve fish with corn salad and charred lime to squeeze over the fish.

NON-FAST DAYS

Serve with 1 slice gluten-free multigrain bread per person. 93 cals per serve.

NUTRITION (PER SERVE)

CALS	FAT	SAT FAT	PROTEIN	CARBS
300	9g	2g	34g	16g

○ VEGETARIAN   ○ VEGAN   ● GLUTEN FREE   ● MAKE AHEAD   ● FREEZABLE

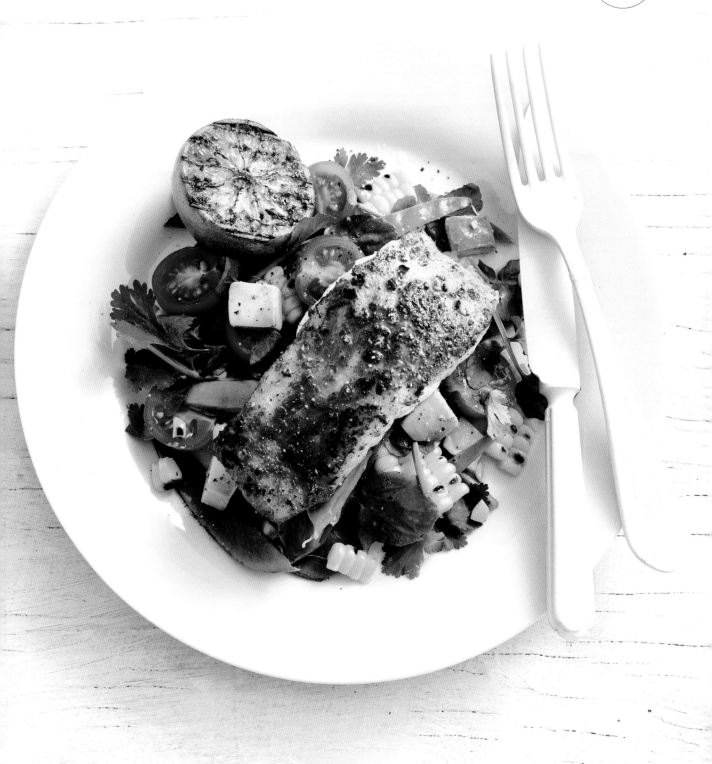

SUMMER VEG LASAGNE

The creamy cottage cheese filling is the star of this impressive vegetarian meal that is packed with vitamins.

SERVES 6 **PREP** 45 mins (+ overnight chilling) **COOK** 20 mins

1 large red capsicum, deseeded, halved
1 large yellow capsicum, deseeded, halved
3 large zucchini, cut lengthways into 5mm slices
1 small eggplant, cut crossways into 5mm discs
2 bunches asparagus, trimmed
4 fresh gluten-free lasagne sheets
400g cottage cheese
2 tsp salted baby capers, rinsed, chopped
2 tsp finely grated lemon rind
2 tbs chopped fresh continental parsley
½ cup fresh basil leaves
Baby beetroot leaves, to serve
6 slices wholegrain gluten-free bread, toasted)

1 Heat a chargrill pan over high heat. Spray capsicum with oil. Grill for 6-8 minutes, until skin is blackened. Transfer to a bowl. Cover. Set aside for 10 minutes to cool. Peel off skin.

2 Meanwhile, spray zucchini and eggplant with oil. Grill for 2-3 minutes each side, until tender. Steam asparagus until tender crisp. Cool.

3 Cook the lasagne in a large saucepan of salted boiling water for 2-3 minutes, until tender. Drain. Combine the cottage cheese, capers and lemon rind in a large bowl.

4 Line an 11 x 21cm (base measurement) loaf pan with plastic wrap, allowing sides to overhang. Line the pan with zucchini, overlapping and allowing 3-4cm to overhang. Layer with yellow capsicum, half the cheese mixture, half the lasagne, the asparagus, eggplant, remaining lasagne, remaining cheese mixture, herbs and red capsicum. Cover with overhanging zucchini, then plastic wrap. Top with cans of food to weight down. Place in fridge overnight to set.

5 To serve, invert and remove plastic wrap. Top with beetroot leaves. Serve with the wholegrain toast.

NUTRITION (PER SERVE)

CALS	FAT	SAT FAT	PROTEIN	CARBS
265	9g	2g	16g	24g

● VEGETARIAN ○ VEGAN ● GLUTEN FREE ● MAKE AHEAD ○ FREEZABLE

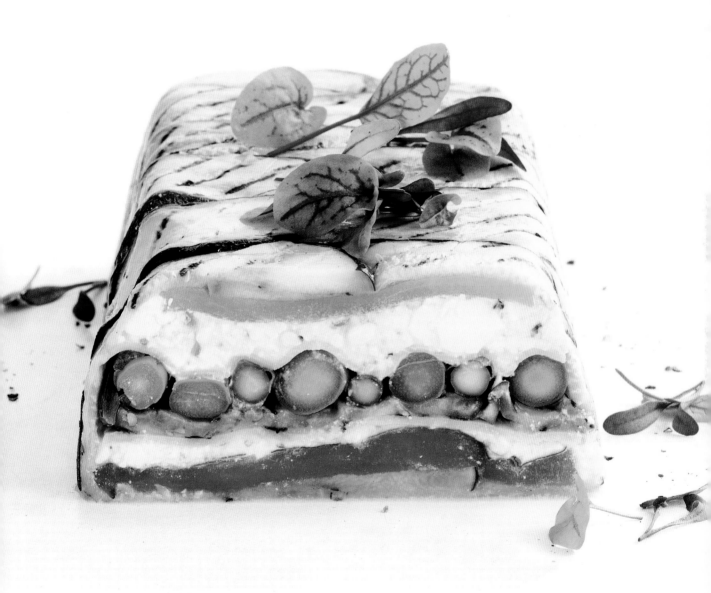

EASY SALAD WITH ROAST
BEEF

This simple salad is packed with iron and protein thanks to the beef, as well as plenty of vegies for added fibre.

SERVES 4 **PREP** 15 mins (+ 10 mins resting) **COOK** 25 mins

2 tsp chopped fresh thyme
1 tsp brown sugar
½ tsp ground cinnamon
1½ tsp smoked paprika
600g lean beef rump roast,
   fat trimmed
2 bunches asparagus, trimmed
2 zucchini, cut crossways into
   1cm slices
2 large vine-ripened tomatoes,
   deseeded, finely chopped
2 tbs chopped fresh
   continental parsley
1 tbs chopped roasted
   unsalted almonds
Pinch of dried chilli flakes
2 tsp fresh lemon juice
2 tsp olive oil
100g mixed salad leaves

1 Preheat oven to 210°C/190°C fan forced. Line a baking tray with baking paper. Combine the thyme, sugar, cinnamon and 1 tsp paprika in a bowl. Rub over the beef. Lightly spray the beef with oil.

2 Heat a large frying pan over high heat. Cook the beef for 1-2 minutes each side or until browned. Transfer to the prepared tray. Roast for 20-25 minutes or until cooked to your liking. Transfer to a plate, cover with foil and set aside for 10 minutes to rest.

3 Meanwhile, heat a barbecue plate or chargrill pan over medium-high heat. Lightly spray the asparagus and zucchini with oil. Grill for 1-2 minutes each side or until tender.

4 Combine tomato, parsley, almonds, chilli flakes, lemon juice, olive oil and remaining ½ tsp paprika in a bowl. Season.

5 Thinly slice the beef. Serve salad leaves, vegies and beef drizzled with dressing.

NON-FAST DAYS

Add 500g boiled and halved baby potatoes to the salad. 84 cals per serve.

NUTRITION (PER SERVE)

CALS	FAT	SAT FAT	PROTEIN	CARBS
290	13g	3g	33g	8g

○ VEGETARIAN   ○ VEGAN   ● **GLUTEN FREE**   ○ MAKE AHEAD   ○ FREEZABLE

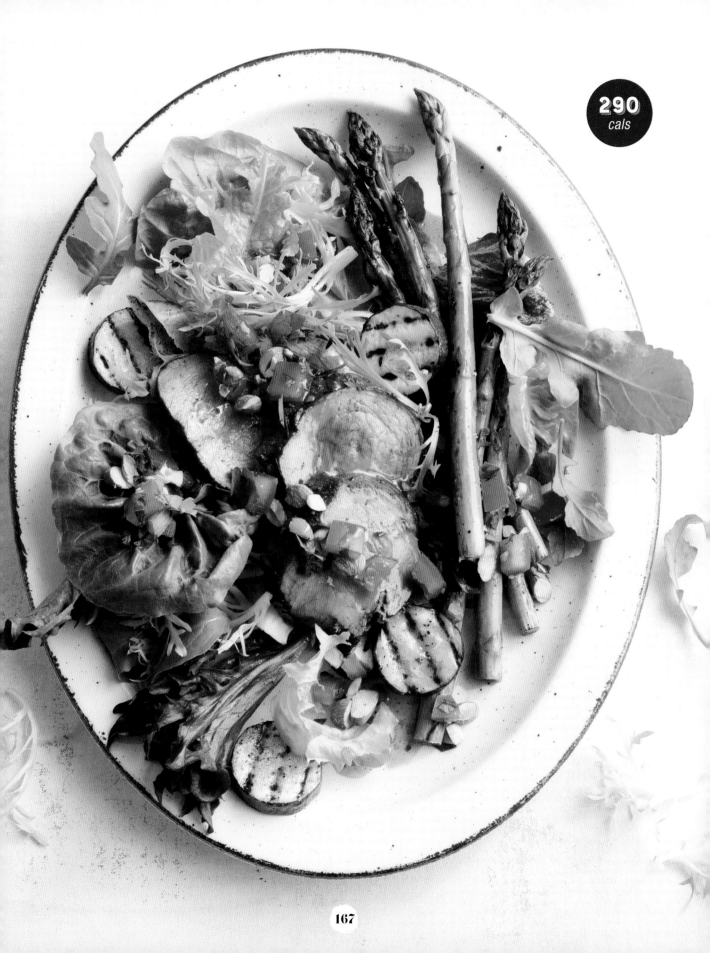

290
cals

SPICY AVO MUFFIN WITH HAM

Enjoy this spicy twist on a favourite Aussie breakfast – ready in five minutes for instant gratification.

SERVES 1 **PREP** 5 mins **COOK** 5 mins

2 tbs avocado
Tabasco sauce, to taste
1 wholegrain English muffin,
   split, toasted
30g shaved salt-reduced lean
   leg ham
20g baby spinach
5 cherry tomatoes, halved

1 Mash avocado in a small bowl. Stir in Tabasco. Season. Spread over muffin halves. Top with ham, spinach and tomato.

NUTRITION (PER SERVE)

CALS	FAT	SAT FAT	PROTEIN	CARBS
263	9g	2g	13g	28g

NON-FAST DAYS

Add a poached egg for an extra protein boost. 65 cals per serve.

★★★★★

A nice quick and easy breakfast for when you don't have much time in the mornings. Kids love it and it also makes a great snack for the afternoon. **HELENB1978**

○ VEGETARIAN   ○ VEGAN   ○ GLUTEN FREE   ○ MAKE AHEAD   ○ FREEZABLE

263
cals

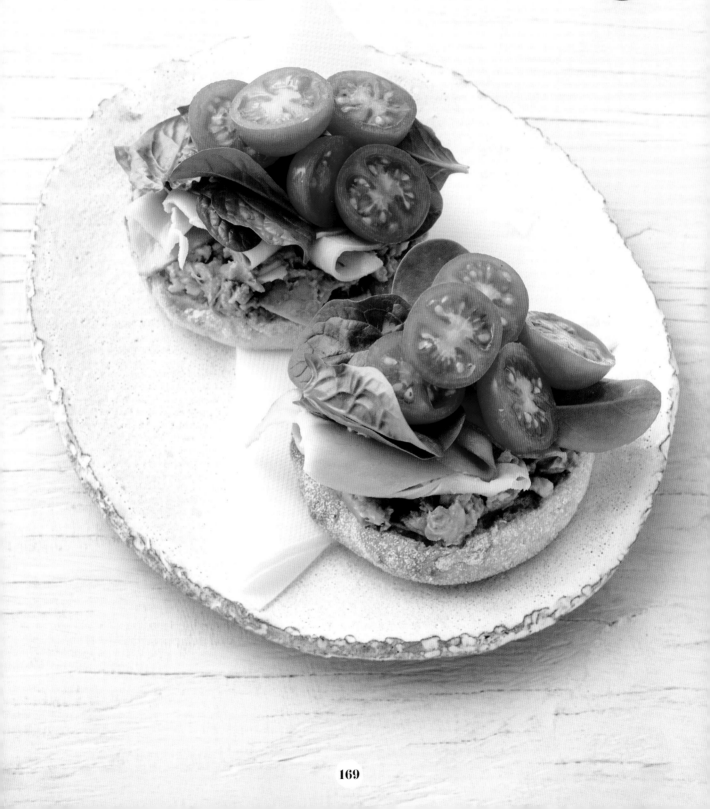

SPEEDY SOBA NOODLE SALAD

This 15-minute Asian noodle salad includes lemon juice to make it a refreshing and tangy side or light lunch.

SERVES 4 **PREP** 10 mins **COOK** 5 mins

180g dried soba noodles
60ml (¼ cup) salt-reduced soy sauce
2 tbs fresh lemon juice
2 tsp sesame oil
½ tsp caster sugar
1 small garlic clove, crushed
1 large Lebanese cucumber, thinly sliced
4 red radishes, trimmed, thinly sliced
3 green shallots, thinly sliced
2 tbs drained pickled ginger
Toasted sesame seeds, to serve

1 Cook noodles in a large saucepan of boiling water, following packet directions. Drain well. Refresh under cold running water. Drain well. Place in a large bowl.

2 Place soy sauce, lemon juice, sesame oil, sugar and garlic in a small bowl. Whisk with a fork to combine. Add cucumber, radish, shallot and dressing to noodles. Toss to combine. Transfer to a serving bowl. Top with pickled ginger. Sprinkle with sesame seeds. Serve.

NON-FAST DAYS

Add 200g chopped Japanese marinated tofu for extra protein. 90 cals per serve.

NUTRITION (PER SERVE)

CALS	FAT	SAT FAT	PROTEIN	CARBS
206	3.4g	0.5g	6.6g	34.7g

Nutrition tip *Toss 100g baby spinach or mixed salad leaves through this salad to increase the vegie count while adding negligible calories. Choose salt-reduced soy sauce to keep sodium levels down.*

CHRISSY FREER

● VEGETARIAN ○ VEGAN ○ GLUTEN FREE ○ MAKE AHEAD ○ FREEZABLE

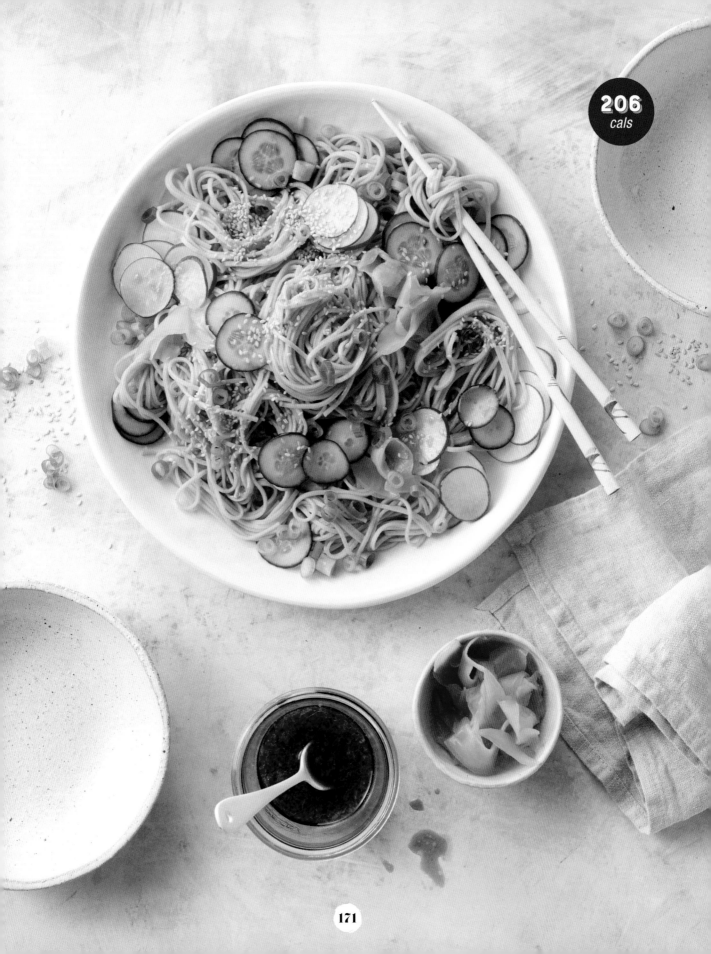

206
cals

BROCCOLI & LEMON SOUP

Packed with green vegies, quinoa and topped with crumbled feta, this super soup is perfect for a midweek meal.

SERVES 4 **PREP** 10 mins **COOK** 20 mins

70g (⅓ cup) tricoloured quinoa
1 tbs extra virgin olive oil
1 brown onion, finely chopped
2 garlic cloves, crushed
2 (about 300g) potatoes, peeled, chopped
1 large head (about 480g) broccoli, stems & florets separated
1L (4 cups) salt-reduced, gluten-free chicken stock
100g baby spinach
½ cup fresh mint leaves
2 tbs fresh lemon juice
2 tsp finely grated lemon rind
80g reduced-fat smooth feta, crumbled
Baby herbs, to serve

1 Place quinoa and 150ml water in a saucepan over high heat. Bring to the boil. Reduce heat to low. Cook, covered, stirring occasionally, for 10-12 minutes or until just tender. Drain and refresh under cold running water.

2 Meanwhile, heat half the oil in a saucepan over medium heat. Add the onion and garlic. Cook, stirring, for 3 minutes or until soft. Stir in the potato and broccoli stems. Add stock and a further 100ml water. Bring to the boil over high heat. Reduce heat to medium and simmer for 10 minutes or until potato is almost soft. Add broccoli florets. Simmer for 6 minutes or until just tender. Add the spinach and mint. Simmer for 1 minute until wilted. Use a stick blender to process until smooth. Stir in lemon juice. Season.

3 Divide soup among bowls. Top with quinoa, lemon rind, feta and baby herbs. Drizzle with remaining oil.

NON-FAST DAYS

Serve with 1 slice gluten-free multigrain bread per person.
93 cals per serve.

NUTRITION (PER SERVE)

CALS	FAT	SAT FAT	PROTEIN	CARBS
277	12g	3g	16g	22g

● VEGETARIAN ○ VEGAN ● GLUTEN FREE ● MAKE AHEAD ● FREEZABLE

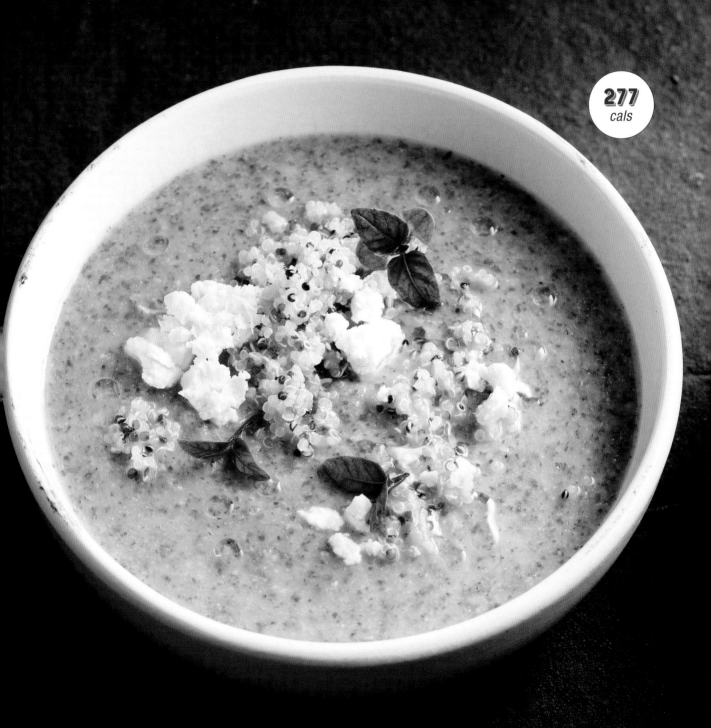

277
cals

★★★★★
My husband and I love this soup; the lemon gives
it a nice kick. I make a double batch so I can freeze
the rest for busy night dinners. JAASMA

WASABI BEEF & ZOODLE SALAD

The wasabi gives this warm salad a great kick, while the combination of fresh flavours and colours make it a memorable meal.

SERVES 4 **PREP** 15 mins (+ 30 mins marinating) **COOK** 10 mins

1 tsp wasabi paste
2 tbs salt-reduced tamari
1½ tbs mirin
2 x 250g lean rump steaks, fat trimmed
145g (1 cup) frozen shelled edamame
250g pkt zucchini noodles
100g baby spinach
1 small red capsicum, deseeded, thinly sliced
½ small red onion, cut into thin wedges
2 tsp sesame seeds, toasted

1 Combine wasabi, tamari and mirin in a small bowl. Place half the dressing in a shallow dish and add the beef. Turn to coat. Cover and set aside for 30 minutes to marinate. Reserve the remaining dressing.

2 Preheat a chargrill pan or barbecue grill over high. Lightly spray beef with oil. Cook beef for 2-3 minutes each side for medium-rare. Transfer to a plate. Cover loosely with foil and set aside for 5 minutes to rest before thinly slicing.

3 Meanwhile, steam edamame for 2-3 minutes over a saucepan of simmering water, adding the zucchini in the last minute of cooking. Drain.

4 Combine the zucchini, edamame, spinach, capsicum and onion in a large serving bowl. Top with the beef and drizzle over the reserved dressing. Sprinkle with sesame seeds.

NUTRITION (PER SERVE)

CALS	FAT	SAT FAT	PROTEIN	CARBS
269	10g	3g	30g	9g

★★★★★ *The marinated beef is delicious – my whole family loved it, which pretty much makes this a miracle recipe!* **CAMSTAR**

○ VEGETARIAN ○ VEGAN ○ GLUTEN FREE ○ MAKE AHEAD ○ FREEZABLE

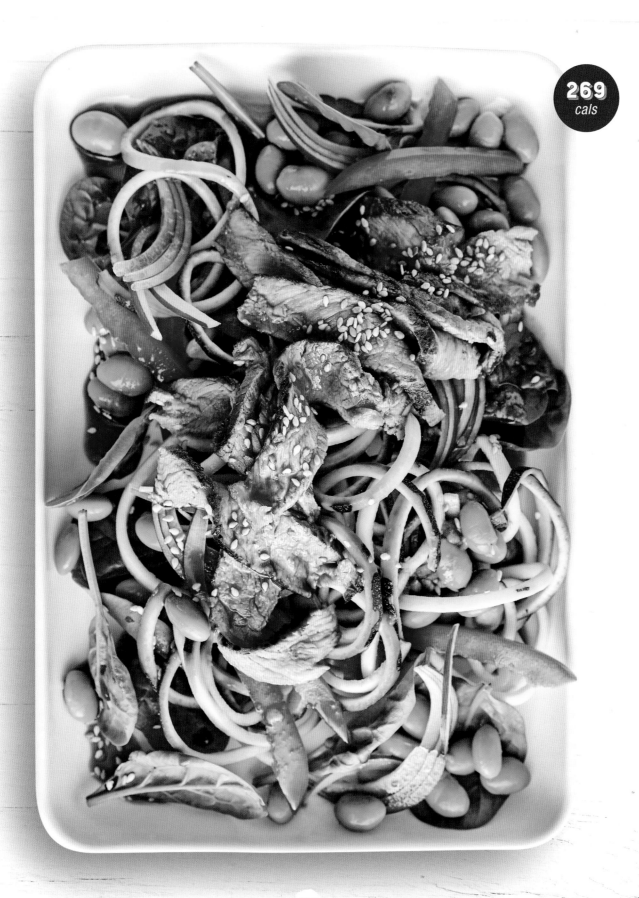

269
cals

EGG WITH AVOCADO &
KALE

This easy (and super-fast) high-protein, low-cal meal
is ideal for breakfast, brunch or even a light lunch.

SERVES 2 **PREP** 10 mins **COOK** 5 mins

1 garlic clove, crushed
100g trimmed kale, washed,
   chopped
2 slices wholegrain bread, toasted
2 eggs, poached
½ small avocado, sliced
Baby herbs, to serve

1 Spray a large non-stick frying pan with oil and heat
over medium-high heat. Add the garlic and cook for
30 seconds or until aromatic.

2 Add kale and cook, stirring, for 2-3 minutes or until
wilted. Divide toast among plates. Top each with wilted
kale, poached egg and ¼ sliced small avocado. Sprinkle with
baby herbs. Season with freshly ground black pepper.

NON-FAST DAYS

To boost protein
and healthy fats,
increase eggs to
2 per serve and
use 1 small
avocado.
100 cals per serve.

NUTRITION (PER SERVE)

CALS	FAT	SAT FAT	PROTEIN	CARBS
238	14g	4g	11g	14g

Nutrition tip

*Kale is a nutritional superstar. Just half a cup of
cooked kale contains 100% of your RDI for vitamin C,
an essential oxidant that aids your body's immune defences
and strengthens resistance to infection.* **CHRISSY FREER**

● **VEGETARIAN** ○ VEGAN ○ GLUTEN FREE ○ MAKE AHEAD ○ FREEZABLE

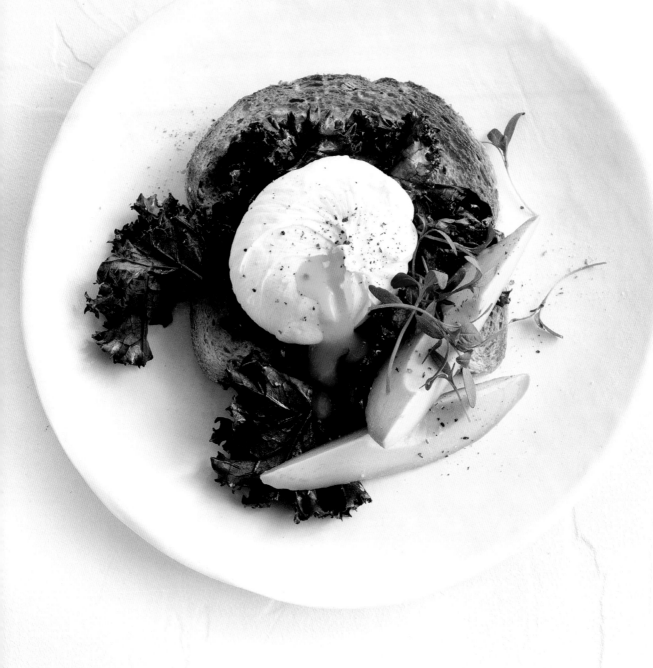

PISTACHIO & QUINOA WITH
BERRIES

Brighten up the morning meal with this bowl of berry bliss – it's quick, easy and gluten-free!

SERVES 1 **PREP** 5 mins **COOK** 5 mins

80g (½ cup) cooked quinoa
½ tsp ground cinnamon
80ml (⅓ cup) cranberry juice
90g (⅓ cup) natural yoghurt
60g (½ cup) fresh berries, to serve
2 tsp chopped pistachios, to serve

1 Combine quinoa, cinnamon, cranberry juice and 2 tbs water in a small saucepan. Bring to the boil over medium heat. Reduce heat and simmer for 2-3 minutes or until liquid is almost absorbed.

2 Spoon the quinoa mixture into a bowl and top with yoghurt. Sprinkle with berries and pistachios.

NON-FAST DAYS

Add a sliced banana to the berries for increased energy levels. 94 cals.

NUTRITION (PER SERVE)

CALS	FAT	SAT FAT	PROTEIN	CARBS
242	7.5g	2.7g	9g	31.2g

Nutrition tip

Cooked quinoa makes a delicious and high-protein breakfast grain. It contains all 9 essential amino acids, making it a rare complete vegetable protein source, ideal for vegetarians. **CHRISSY FREER**

● VEGETARIAN ○ VEGAN ● GLUTEN FREE ○ MAKE AHEAD ○ FREEZABLE

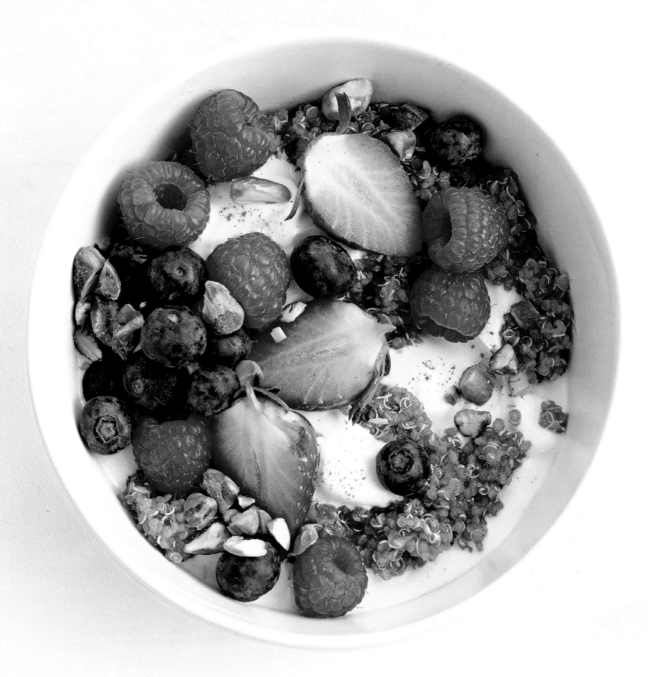

ZUCCHINI SALAD WITH CHILLI

Asian flavours, including mint and coriander, combine with ginger and tamari to create this no-cook salad with extra crunch.

SERVES 4 **PREP** 15 mins

4 large zucchini, trimmed
2 corncobs, husks and
   silk removed
250g cherry tomatoes, halved
⅓ cup fresh mint leaves
⅓ cup fresh coriander leaves
1 long fresh red chilli, deseeded,
   finely chopped
1 tbs fresh lime juice
2 tsp salt-reduced gluten-free tamari
1 tsp finely grated fresh ginger
1 tsp caster sugar
45g (¼ cup) coarsely chopped
   roasted unsalted cashews

1 Cut the zucchini into long strands using a spiraliser, stopping when you reach the seeds. Alternatively, cut the zucchini into long ribbons using a vegetable peeler. Use a sharp knife to cut the kernels from the corn.

2 Combine the zucchini, corn, tomato, mint and coriander in a large bowl. Combine the chilli, lime juice, tamari, ginger and sugar in a small bowl. Stir to dissolve the sugar.

3 Drizzle the dressing over the salad and toss gently to combine. Serve scattered with the cashews.

NON-FAST DAYS

To boost protein toss a 400g can rinsed and drained chickpeas through salad. 68 cals per serve.

NUTRITION (PER SERVE)

CALS	FAT	SAT FAT	PROTEIN	CARBS
179	9g	1g	6g	14g

★★★★★

Delicious! Made it last night exactly to recipe and it was divine! Will definitely be having again. The flavours were perfect. **DEBINBRIS**

● VEGETARIAN ● VEGAN ● GLUTEN FREE ○ MAKE AHEAD ○ FREEZABLE

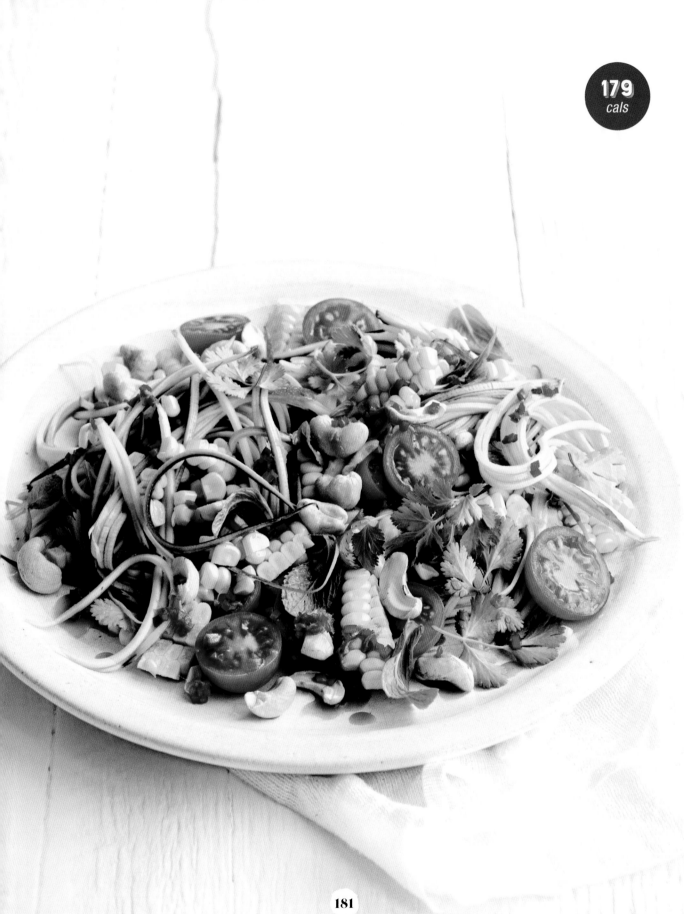

179
cals

LIME & LEMONGRASS
CHICKEN

These zesty lettuce wraps make for a refreshing light meal or lunch – perfect for hot summer days.

SERVES 4 **PREP** 10 mins (+ 10 mins marinating) **COOK** 15 mins

1 stem lemongrass, pale section only, finely chopped
2 tsp finely grated lime rind
2 tsp macadamia or sunflower oil
500g chicken breast fillets, thinly sliced
100g sweet potato noodles (assi dangmyeon)
¼ red cabbage, shredded
2 carrots, peeled, cut into matchsticks
110g (2 cups) trimmed bean sprouts
1 tbs fresh lime juice
2 tsp salt-reduced gluten-free tamari
1 small fresh red chilli, deseeded, finely chopped
1 tsp brown sugar
8 iceberg lettuce leaves
Fresh mint leaves, to serve

1 Combine the lemongrass, lime rind and oil in a shallow glass or ceramic dish. Add the chicken and toss to coat. Cover and set aside for 10 minutes to marinate.

2 Meanwhile, cook the noodles following packet directions or until al dente. Drain.

3 Heat a large wok over high heat. Stir-fry the chicken, in 2 batches, for 5 minutes or until cooked through. Transfer to a bowl. Spray the wok with a little oil. Stir-fry the cabbage and carrot over medium-high heat for 2 minutes. Add the bean sprouts and stir-fry for 1 minute.

4 Combine the lime juice, tamari, chilli and sugar in a small bowl. Stir until sugar dissolves. Place the noodles, vegetables and chicken in a bowl. Toss to combine. Divide among lettuce leaves. Top with mint leaves and drizzle with lime dressing.

COOK'S NOTE

For a dose of healthy fats, add ⅓ cup roasted chopped cashew nuts to the noodles. 59 cals per serve.

NUTRITION (PER SERVE)

CALS	FAT	SAT FAT	PROTEIN	CARBS
293	5g	1g	31g	28g

○ VEGETARIAN ○ VEGAN ● GLUTEN FREE ○ MAKE AHEAD ○ FREEZABLE

293
cals

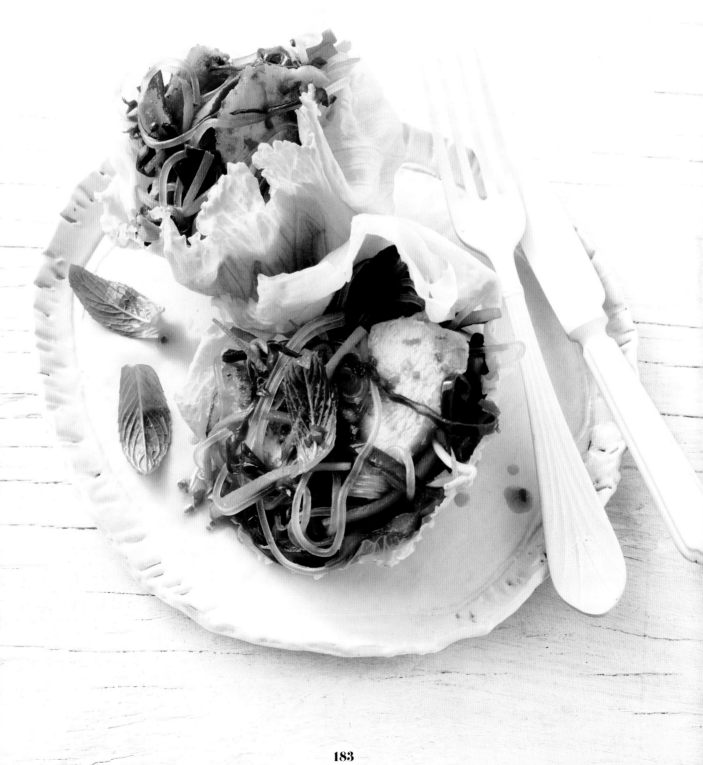

NUTTY COFFEE GRANOLA

Skip your morning latte and get your coffee fix with this aromatic granola full of nuts and spices.

SERVES 12 **PREP** 10 mins (+ cooling) **COOK** 30 mins

270g (3 cups) traditional rolled oats
80g (½ cup) pepitas
145g (1 cup) raw cashews
110g (⅔ cup) skinless hazelnuts
1 tsp ground cinnamon
1 tsp ground ginger
½ tsp mixed spice
60ml (¼ cup) honey
60ml (¼ cup) strong brewed coffee
1 tbs coconut oil, melted
2 tsp vanilla extract
15g (¼ cup) coconut flakes

1 Preheat oven to 180°C/160°C fan forced. Line 2 large baking trays with baking paper.

2 Place oats, pepitas, cashews, hazelnuts, cinnamon, ginger and mixed spice in a large bowl. Toss to combine. Divide mixture between prepared trays. Combine honey, coffee, coconut oil and vanilla in a jug. Drizzle over oat mixture on trays. Stir to coat. Sprinkle with a pinch of salt.

3 Bake for 20-25 minutes, stirring twice during cooking. Sprinkle coconut flakes over oat mixture. Bake for 3-4 minutes or until golden. Remove from oven. Set aside to cool completely before storing in an airtight container.

NON-FAST DAYS

Top each serve with 2 tbs natural yoghurt, ½ sliced banana and 2 tbs blueberries. 89 cals per serve.

NUTRITION (GRANOLA ONLY)

CALS	FAT	SAT FAT	PROTEIN	CARBS
296	19.1g	4.3g	8.8g	20.8g

● VEGETARIAN ○ VEGAN ○ GLUTEN FREE ● MAKE AHEAD ○ FREEZABLE

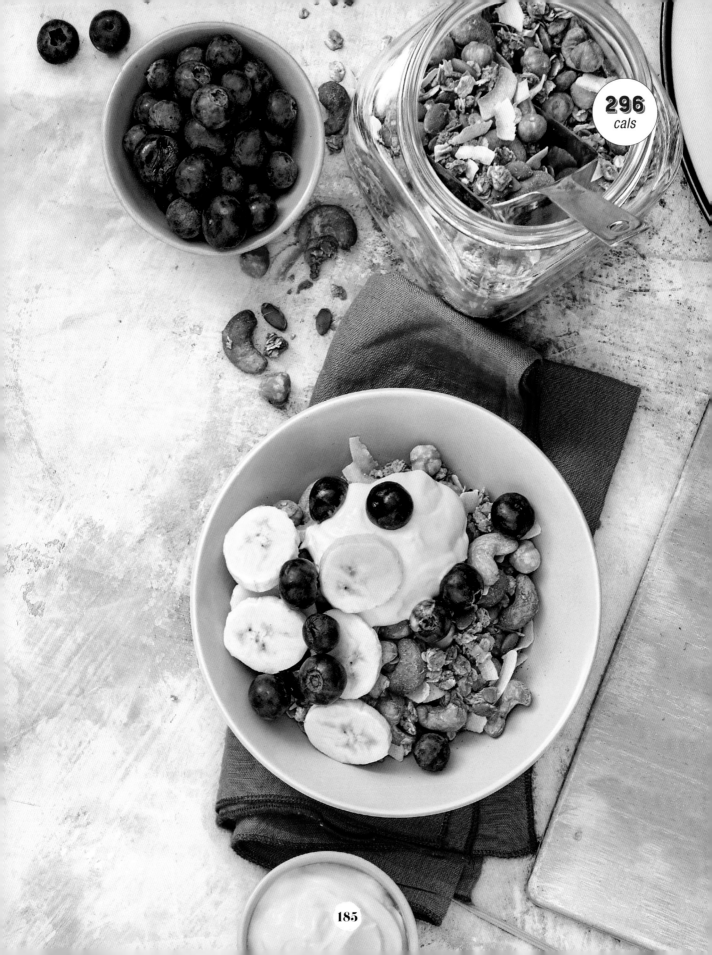

296
cals

SESAME TUNA WITH APPLE SLAW

Nutrient-rich sesame seeds form a delectable and crunchy crust for these tuna steaks that will be on the table in 20 minutes.

SERVES 4 **PREP** 15 mins **COOK** 5 mins

2 tbs sesame seeds
4 (150g each) fresh tuna steaks
¼ small green cabbage, trimmed, shredded
1 large red apple, cored, cut into matchsticks
3 large celery sticks, trimmed, cut into matchsticks
4 small red radishes, trimmed, cut into matchsticks
1 tbs chopped fresh chives
1½ tbs salt-reduced gluten-free soy sauce
1½ tbs fresh lemon juice
½ tsp caster sugar
1 tsp sesame oil
2 tbs pomegranate seeds

1 Place the sesame seeds on a plate. Press 1 side of the tuna into the sesame seeds to coat. Set aside.

2 Place the cabbage, apple, celery, radish and chives in a large bowl. Stir the soy, lemon juice, sugar and sesame oil in a small bowl until sugar dissolves.

3 Heat a large non-stick frying pan over high heat. Spray with olive oil. Cook the tuna, sesame-side down, for 1-2 minutes or until golden. Turn and cook for a further minute for medium, or until cooked to your liking.

4 Divide slaw among plates. Top with the tuna, drizzle with the dressing and scatter with pomegranate seeds.

NON-FAST DAYS

Cook 180g dried 100% buckwheat noodles, if you like. Rinse, drain and toss through salad. 160 cals per serve.

NUTRITION (PER SERVE)

CALS	FAT	SAT FAT	PROTEIN	CARBS
295	7g	1g	45g	11g

○ VEGETARIAN ○ VEGAN ● GLUTEN FREE ○ MAKE AHEAD ○ FREEZABLE

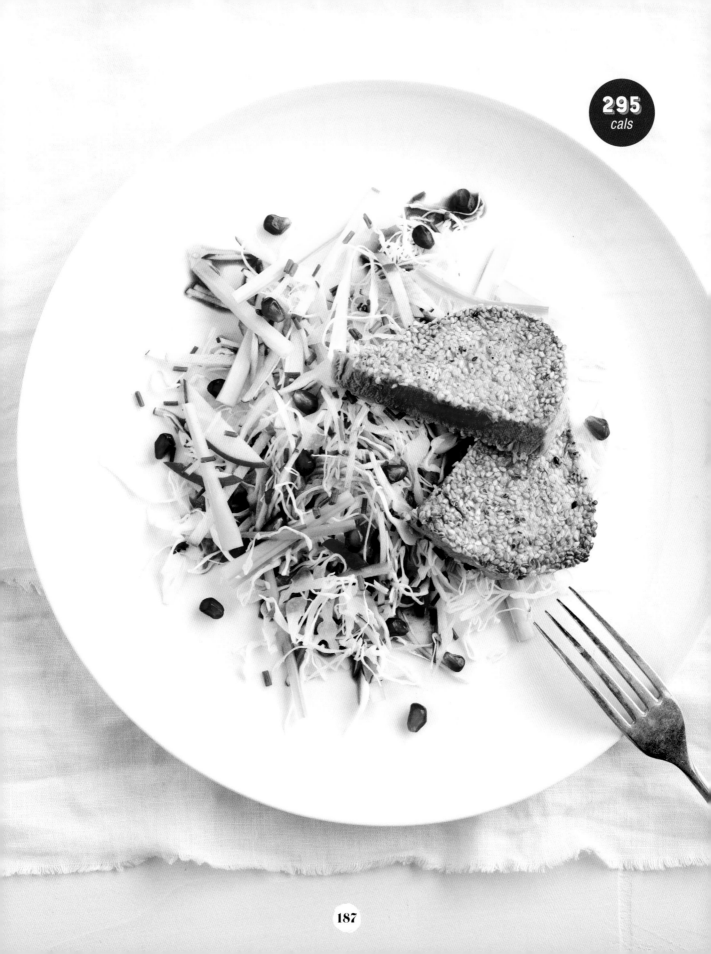

FRITTATA WITH TOMATO &
GREENS

The fresh flavours of this delicious frittata elevate it to the top of the lunch list. Serve with a simple salad for added crunch.

SERVES 4 **PREP** 15 mins **COOK** 35 mins

1 bunch asparagus, trimmed, sliced
200g broccoli, cut into large florets
8 eggs
60ml (¼ cup) milk
2 tbs chopped fresh chives
2 tbs chopped fresh basil
70g creamy feta, crumbled
150g cherry tomatoes, halved, plus
   100g extra, to serve
80g mixed salad leaves, to serve

1 Preheat oven to 180°C/160°C fan forced. Line a 16 x 26cm (base measurement) slice pan with baking paper.

2 Place the asparagus and broccoli in a steamer over a saucepan of simmering water. Cover and steam for 2 minutes or until tender crisp. Refresh under cold running water. Drain. Coarsely chop broccoli.

3 Whisk eggs, milk, herbs and two-thirds of the feta in a large bowl. Add steamed vegetables and stir to combine. Pour into prepared pan. Arrange tomato halves and remaining feta over the top.

4 Bake for 25-30 minutes or until golden, puffed and set in the middle. Set aside to cool. Cut into pieces. Serve with salad leaves and extra tomato.

NON-FAST DAYS

Add 1 cup cooked quinoa in step 3 and drizzle the salad with 1 tbs extra virgin olive oil and 2 tsp balsamic vinegar. 80 cals per serve.

NUTRITION (PER SERVE)

CALS	FAT	SAT FAT	PROTEIN	CARBS
230	14g	5g	21g	4g

● VEGETARIAN   ○ VEGAN   ● GLUTEN FREE   ● MAKE AHEAD   ○ FREEZABLE

★★★★★ *Super easy to make, I added ham and it was delicious. Also microwaved the vegies to make it faster (and less to clean up).* **SHIRL1545**

230 cals

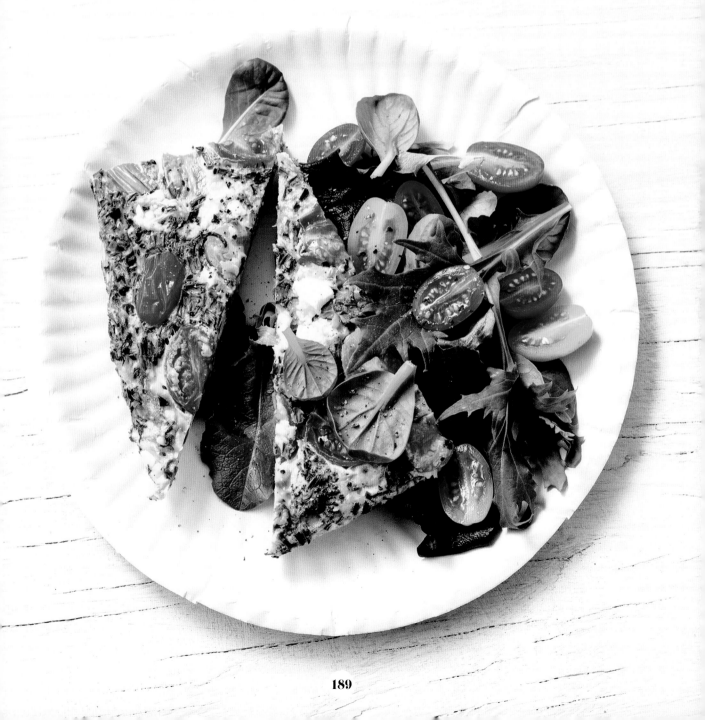

HASH BROWN & EGG
CUPS

This fun (and fast) breakfast idea is guaranteed to be popular with the whole family.

MAKES 8 **PREP** 15 mins (+ 5 mins standing) **COOK** 25 mins

600g cream delight potatoes, peeled, finely grated
50g (⅔ cup) finely grated parmesan
3 rashers streaky bacon, finely chopped
1 tbs chopped fresh chives
8 small eggs

1 Preheat oven to 200°C/180°C fan forced. Grease 8 holes of a 12-hole (⅓-cup capacity) muffin pan.

2 Squeeze excess moisture from potato. Pat dry with paper towel. Combine potato and parmesan in a bowl. Season. Divide potato mixture evenly among holes in prepared pan. Using the back of a teaspoon, press mixture evenly over base and side of holes to form a case. Bake for 15 minutes or until potato is golden.

3 Sprinkle half of the bacon and half the chives over the base of each case. Crack 1 egg into each hole. Sprinkle with remaining bacon and chives. Bake for 10 minutes or until egg is just set and bacon is golden. Stand in pans for 5 minutes. Carefully transfer to a baking paper-lined wire rack to cool. Serve warm or cold.

NON-FAST DAYS

Serve with 1 slice (38g) gluten-free multigrain bread topped with ¼ small avocado per person. 148 cals per serve.

NUTRITION (EACH)

CALS	FAT	SAT FAT	PROTEIN	CARBS
175	10.3g	4.2g	11.7g	8.5g

○ VEGETARIAN ○ VEGAN ● GLUTEN FREE ○ MAKE AHEAD ○ FREEZABLE

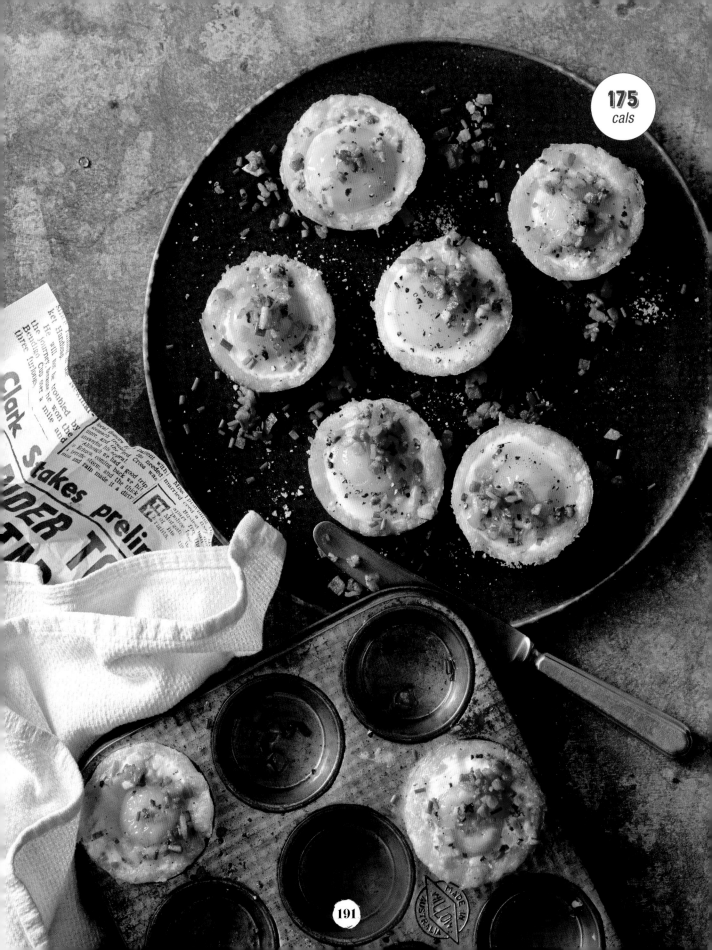

175
cals

SAN CHOY BAU
BOWL

Turn san choy bau into a quick healthy dinner bowl by swapping pork mince for lean chicken mince and adding lots of vegies.

SERVES 4 **PREP** 15 mins **COOK** 10 mins

2 tsp sesame oil
1 onion, finely chopped
2 celery sticks, finely chopped
2 garlic cloves, crushed
2 tsp finely grated fresh ginger
500g lean chicken breast mince
225g can water chestnuts, drained, finely chopped
1 tbs gluten-free oyster sauce
1 tbs salt-reduced gluten-free tamari
2 baby gem lettuces, trimmed, leaves separated
1 Lebanese cucumber, thinly sliced
1 large carrot, peeled, shredded
110g (2 cups) trimmed bean sprouts
Fresh coriander leaves and sliced red chilli, to serve

1 Heat the oil in a large wok over high heat. Stir-fry the onion and celery for 2 minutes or until softened. Add the garlic and ginger and stir-fry for 1 minute or until aromatic. Add the mince and stir-fry, breaking mince up with a wooden spoon, for 3-4 minutes or until golden. Add the water chestnuts, oyster sauce and tamari and stir-fry for 1 minute or until heated through.

2 Divide lettuce leaves, mince mixture, cucumber, carrot and bean sprouts among serving bowls. Serve topped with coriander and chilli.

NON-FAST DAYS

Serve with ½ cup steamed brown rice per person. 138 cals per serve.

NUTRITION (PER SERVE)

CALS	FAT	SAT FAT	PROTEIN	CARBS
272	13g	4g	25g	9g

★★★★★ *Quick, easy, full of flavour and the whole family loved it. Recommend you give it a try – it will become one of the family favourites.* **PRATTYSKHALEESI**

○ VEGETARIAN ○ VEGAN ● GLUTEN FREE ○ MAKE AHEAD ○ FREEZABLE

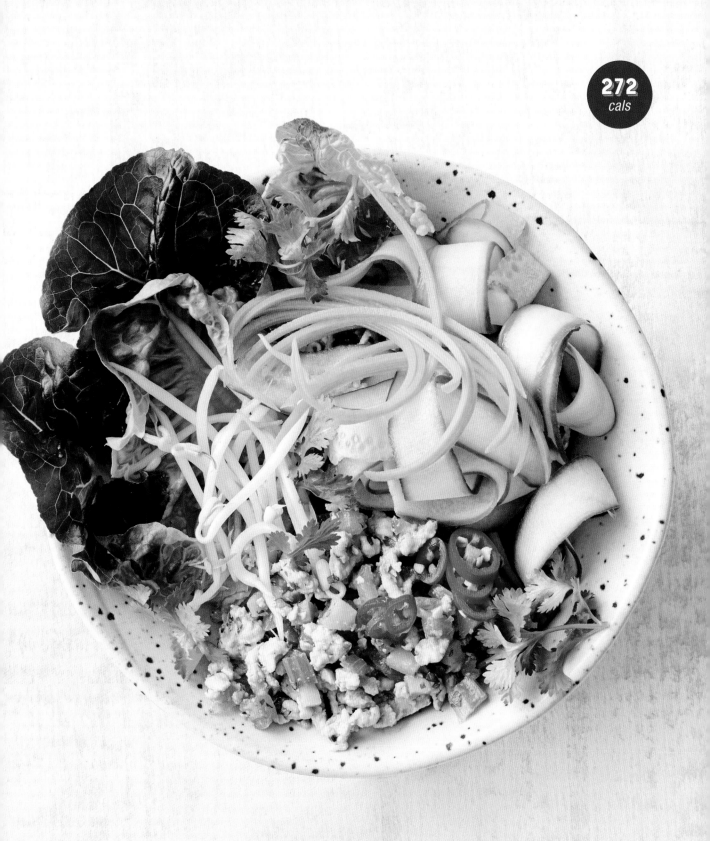

272
cals

193

CHEESY LUNCHBOX
OMELETTE
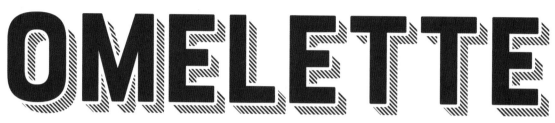

Tick all the boxes with this vegetarian, low-cal, low-fat, gluten-free and nutritious omelette, perfect for school lunches.

SERVES 6 **PREP** 10 mins **COOK** 40 mins

1 tbs extra virgin olive oil
250g pkt sweet potato noodles
250g pkt zucchini noodles, drained
2 tomatoes, chopped
2 garlic cloves, finely chopped
2 green shallots, trimmed,
    thinly sliced
½ cup shredded fresh basil leaves,
    plus extra leaves, to serve
8 large eggs
20g (¼ cup) finely grated parmesan
125g feta, cut into thin slices, halved
1 tbs pepitas
Grape tomatoes (optional), to serve

1 Heat the oil in a 19cm base measurement (24cm top measurement) ovenproof frying pan over medium-high heat. Add the sweet potato noodles to the pan and cook, stirring often, for 8 minutes or until softened. Add the zucchini to the pan and cook, stirring often, for 3-5 minutes or until the sweet potato is tender. Add the tomatoes, garlic and shallot and cook for a further 2 minutes. Stir in the basil. Use a slotted spoon to transfer to a bowl.

2 Preheat the oven to 170°C/150°C fan forced. Whisk together the eggs with 2 tbs water. Season. Stir through half of the parmesan. Pour the egg mixture into the frying pan. Top with the noodle mixture. Arrange the feta on top. Sprinkle with pepitas and remaining parmesan. Cook on the stove top for 5 minutes. Transfer to the oven and cook for 15-20 minutes, or until the eggs are set. Serve with extra basil leaves and grape tomatoes, if you like.

NON-FAST DAYS

Serve with 1 slice gluten-free multigrain bread per person. 93 cals per serve.

NUTRITION (PER SERVE)

CALS	FAT	SAT FAT	PROTEIN	CARBS
147	9g	4g	7g	8g

● VEGETARIAN ○ VEGAN ● GLUTEN FREE ○ MAKE AHEAD ○ FREEZABLE

★★★★★
I enjoyed everything about this! The flavoures were delicious – the fried zucchini and sweet potato, the feta, the tomato. **BELHOP**

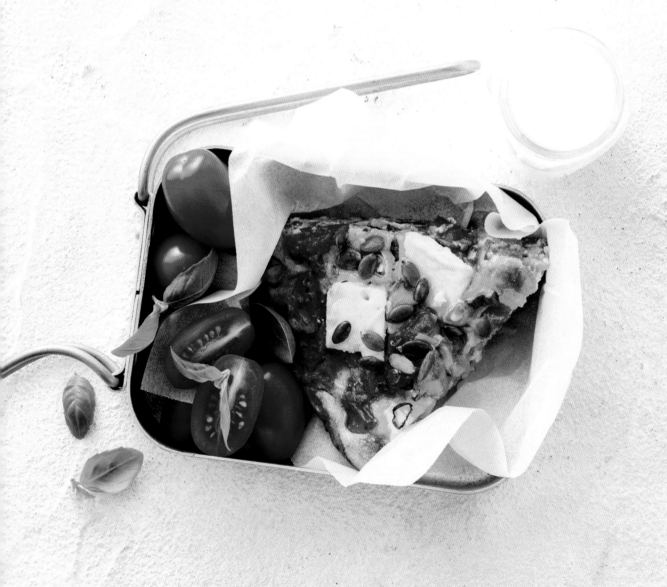

BREAKFAST QUINOA

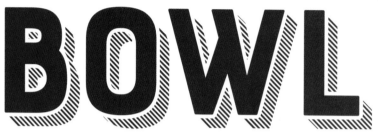

BOWL

A winning combination of fruit, nuts and spices makes this stunning salad perfect for morning meals.

SERVES 4 **PREP** 10 mins **COOK** 15 mins

135g (⅔ cup) quinoa, rinsed, drained
2 navel oranges
½ tsp ground cinnamon, plus extra
   to serve
2 tbs pepitas
2 tbs natural almonds, chopped
125g fresh blueberries
190g (⅔ cup) natural yoghurt,
   to serve

1 Place the quinoa and 330ml (1⅓ cups) water in a saucepan over medium-high heat. Bring to the boil. Reduce heat to low and simmer, covered, for 12 minutes or until the water has evaporated and the quinoa is just tender. Transfer to a large bowl and set aside to cool.

2 Peel and segment the oranges over a bowl, reserving the juice, and add the orange segments, juice, cinnamon, pepitas, almonds and half of the blueberries to the cooked quinoa. Stir to combine.

3 Divide quinoa mixture among bowls. Top with the remaining blueberries. Dollop with yoghurt. Sprinkle with the extra cinnamon.

NON-FAST DAYS

Double the quantity of yoghurt, almonds and pepitas to boost protein. 98 cals per serve.

NUTRITION (PER SERVE)

CALS	FAT	SAT FAT	PROTEIN	CARBS
272	9.5g	2g	10g	32.2g

● VEGETARIAN ○ VEGAN ● GLUTEN FREE ○ MAKE AHEAD ○ FREEZABLE

272
cals

★ ★ ★ ★ ★ *Love this breakfast recipe!
I usually eat mine at 8am and I'm never hungry
before midday.* **ALYSE-GRACE**

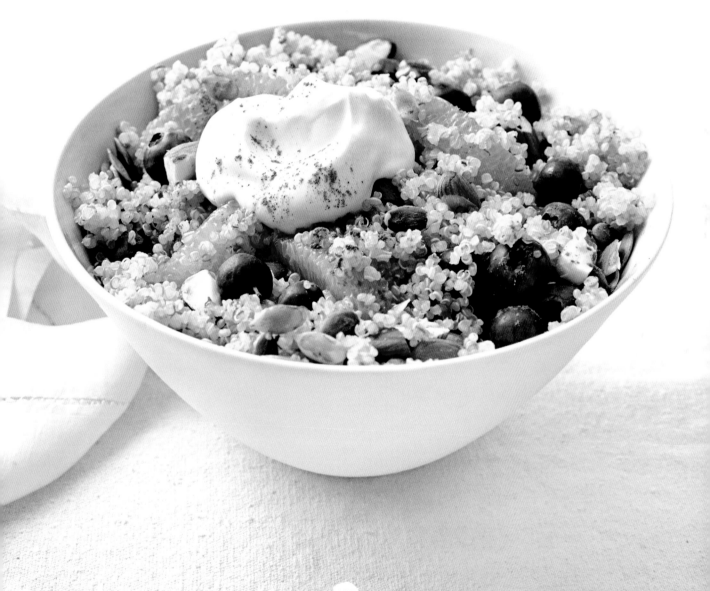

197

SALAD WITH CUCUMBER &

FETA

The generous slice of cheese adds just the right amount of creamy goodness to this simple and speedy salad.

SERVES 4 **PREP** 10 mins (+ 1 hour standing)

2 continental cucumbers, scrubbed, trimmed, halved crossways
1 tbs extra virgin olive oil
2 tsp red wine vinegar
60g kalamata olives
100g cherry tomatoes, halved
1 small red onion, thinly sliced
200g block feta, quartered diagonally
½ tsp dried oregano leaves
Pinch dried chilli flakes

1 Use a vegetable peeler to peel thin strips from the cucumber. Place in a bowl of iced water. Set aside for 1 hour or until curled. Drain and gently pat dry.

2 Meanwhile, whisk the oil and red wine vinegar together in a small bowl and season.

3 Place the cucumber strips, olives, tomato, onion and half the dressing in a bowl. Toss to combine. Place on a serving plate. Top with the feta. Sprinkle the feta with the oregano and chilli. Drizzle with remaining dressing.

NON-FAST DAYS

Add a 400g can chickpeas, rinsed and drained, to the salad for extra protein. 68 cals per serve.

NUTRITION (PER SERVE)

CALS	FAT	SAT FAT	PROTEIN	CARBS
248	19.6g	8.6g	10.5g	4.5g

Nutrition tip *Cucumbers are predominately water and therefore low in calories and fat, making them the perfect food for fasting days. They are also rich in pectin, a soluble fibre that helps to promote gut health.* **CHRISSY FREER**

○ VEGETARIAN   ○ VEGAN   ● GLUTEN FREE   ● MAKE AHEAD   ● FREEZABLE

248
cals

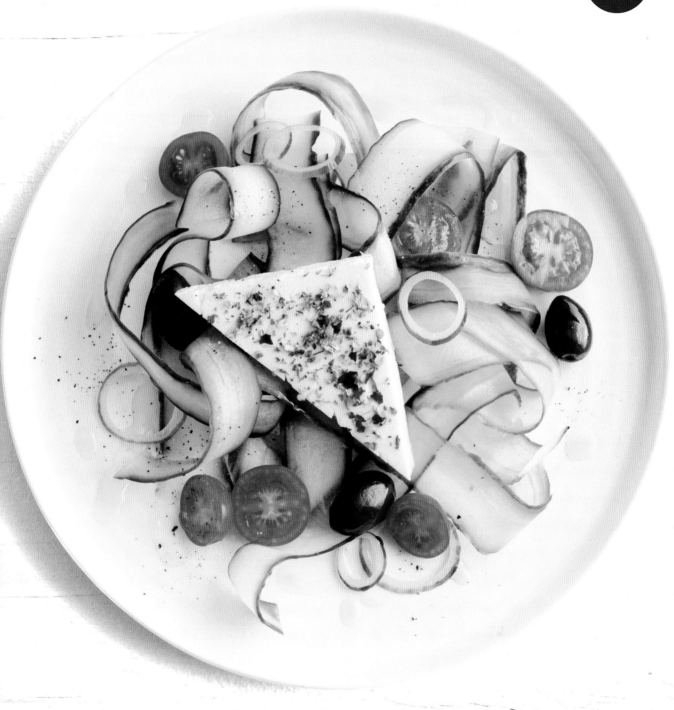

CORN WITH BARBECUED TOFU

The fresh flavours and colourful ingredients in this salad make it ideal for simple lunch or a light meal.

SERVES 4   **PREP** 10 mins   **COOK** 15 mins

2 tsp finely grated lemon rind
1 tsp dried oregano leaves
2 tbs fresh lemon juice
2 tsp extra virgin olive oil
300g firm tofu, drained, cut into
  1cm slices
2 corncobs, husks and
  silk removed
2 bunches asparagus, trimmed
1 tbs basil pesto
100g baby rocket
250g mixed cherry tomatoes, halved
2 tbs shaved parmesan

1. Combine the lemon rind, oregano, 1 tbs lemon juice and 1 tsp olive oil in a small bowl. Brush the oregano mixture evenly over the sliced tofu.

2. Preheat a chargrill pan or barbecue grill over high heat. Lightly spray the tofu, corn and asparagus with oil. Cook the corn for 8 minutes, turning, or until tender. Cook tofu and asparagus for 1-2 minutes each side or until lightly charred and asparagus is tender.

3. Meanwhile, whisk the pesto, remaining 1 tbs lemon juice and 1 tsp olive oil in a small bowl until combined.

4. Cut the corncobs into 1.5cm-thick discs. Combine the corn, rocket, tomato and asparagus in a bowl. Divide among serving plates or place on a large platter. Top with the tofu and drizzle with the pesto dressing. Scatter with parmesan to serve.

NON-FAST DAYS

Add 250g pkt microwave black rice, heated, in step 4.
132 cals per serve.

NUTRITION (PER SERVE)

CALS	FAT	SAT FAT	PROTEIN	CARBS
286	15.8g	3g	16.8g	13.4g

● VEGETARIAN   ○ VEGAN   ● GLUTEN FREE   ○ MAKE AHEAD   ○ FREEZABLE

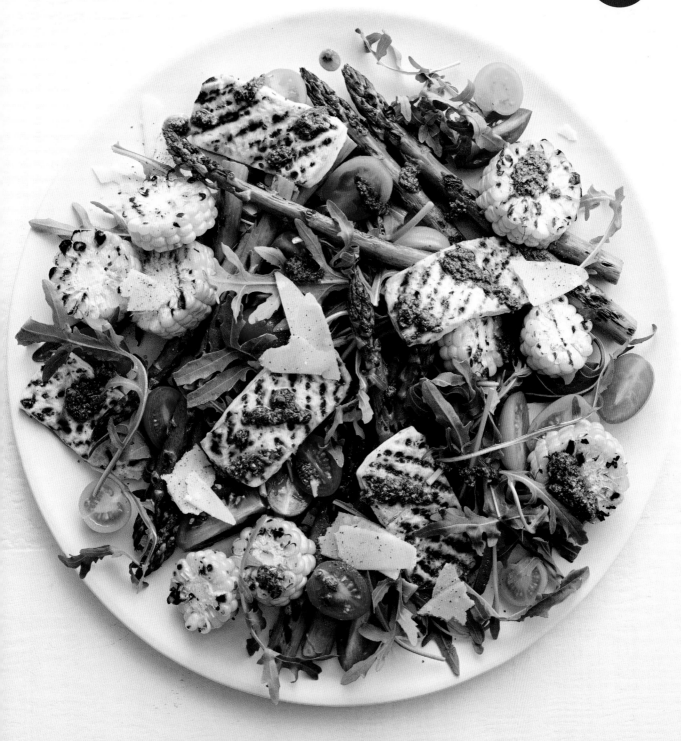

MAKE-AHEAD CHIA & OATS

These healthy overnight oats are prepared in a jar to be even easier to transport. Topped with yoghurt and berries, everyone will love them.

SERVES 4 **PREP** 10 mins (+ overnight soaking)

125g (1⅓ cups) rolled oats
2 tbs chia seeds
2 tbs pepitas
1 tsp ground cinnamon
1 tsp vanilla bean paste
1½ tbs nut butter
1 tbs pure maple syrup
500ml (2 cups) almond coconut milk
130g (½ cup) natural yoghurt
120g fresh or frozen raspberries

1 Combine the oats, chia seeds, pepitas, cinnamon, vanilla, nut butter, maple syrup and almond milk in a large bowl.

2 Divide the oat mixture among 4 jars or bowls. Top each with one-quarter of the yoghurt and berries. Cover and store in the fridge overnight.

NON-FAST DAYS

Top each jar with 2 tbs chopped almonds. 118 cals per serve.

NUTRITION (PER SERVE)

CALS	FAT	SAT FAT	PROTEIN	CARBS
288	13.7g	2.6g	10.4g	26.1g

★★★★★

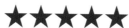

These taste great and are super easy to make. Followed the recipe exactly. **LG22**

● VEGETARIAN ○ VEGAN ○ GLUTEN FREE ● MAKE AHEAD ○ FREEZABLE

288
cals

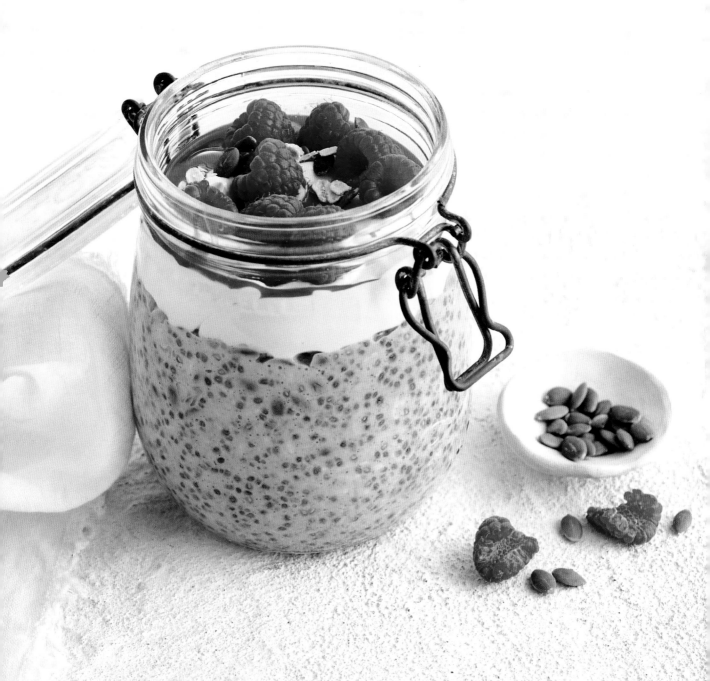

SMASHED AVO ON SWEET POTATO

Swapping the toast for gluten-free sweet potato creates the perfect healthy breakfast for one!

SERVES 1 **PREP** 5 mins **COOK** 10 mins

2 x 5mm-thick slices sweet potato
¼ large avocado
1 tbs fresh ricotta
1 tsp fresh lemon juice
Pinch of dried chilli flakes
20g baby spinach
1 egg, poached, to serve

1 Place sweet potato slices in a toaster and toast until golden and tender (this may take 2-3 cycles).

2 Meanwhile, mash avocado and ricotta together in a small bowl. Stir through lemon juice and chilli flakes.

3 Spread avocado mixture over toasted sweet potato. Top with spinach and a poached egg.

NON-FAST DAYS

Need more protein? Add an extra egg to keep your energy levels up! 65 cals.

NUTRITION (PER SERVE)

CALS	FAT	SAT FAT	PROTEIN	CARBS
253	15g	4g	12g	15g

Nutrition tip

Avocado makes the perfect healthy substitute for butter on toast. Rich in heart-healthy monounsaturated fatty acids, avocados are also a good source of vitamins C, E and B6. **CHRISSY FREER**

● VEGETARIAN ○ VEGAN ● GLUTEN FREE ○ MAKE AHEAD ○ FREEZABLE

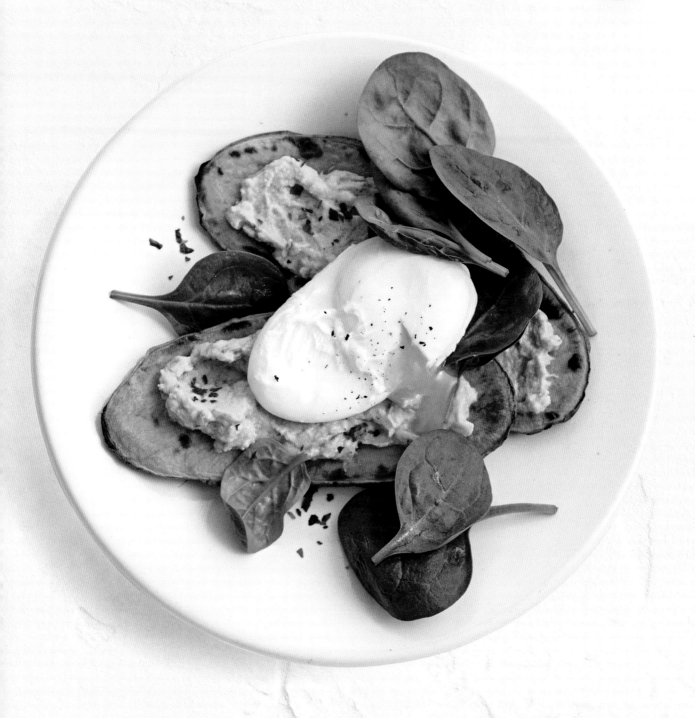

253
cals

SWEET POTATO & LENTIL PATTIES

These easy gluten-free patties are also portable – making them perfect for picnics or office lunch solutions.

SERVES 4 **PREP** 15 mins (+ cooling) **COOK** 45 mins

500g sweet potato, peeled, cut into 2cm cubes
½ tsp ground cumin
½ tsp ground coriander
400g can brown lentils, rinsed, drained
2 tbs chopped fresh coriander
30g (½ cup) fresh wholegrain gluten-free breadcrumbs
2 tsp extra virgin olive oil
85g (⅓ cup) tzatziki
100g baby rocket
200g grape tomatoes, halved

1 Preheat oven to 200°C/180°C fan forced. Line a large baking tray with baking paper. Place potato on prepared tray. Lightly spray with olive oil and sprinkle with cumin and ground coriander. Roast for 25-30 minutes or until tender. Place in a bowl. Coarsely mash. Cool.

2 Add lentils, fresh coriander and breadcrumbs to potato mixture. Stir until well combined. Season. Shape into eight 2cm-thick patties.

3 Heat oil in a large non-stick frying pan over medium-high heat. Cook patties, in batches, for 2-3 minutes each side or until golden. Divide tzatziki among plates. Top with rocket, tomato and patties.

NON-FAST DAYS

Serve in a multigrain gluten-free wrap. 100 cals per serve.

NUTRITION (PER SERVE)

CALS	FAT	SAT FAT	PROTEIN	CARBS
254	6g	1g	11g	35g

★★★★★ *These were very easy to make and tasted really good. Great for a weeknight meat-free meal.* **LITTLEPLUMJ22**

● VEGETARIAN ○ VEGAN ● GLUTEN FREE ○ MAKE AHEAD ○ FREEZABLE

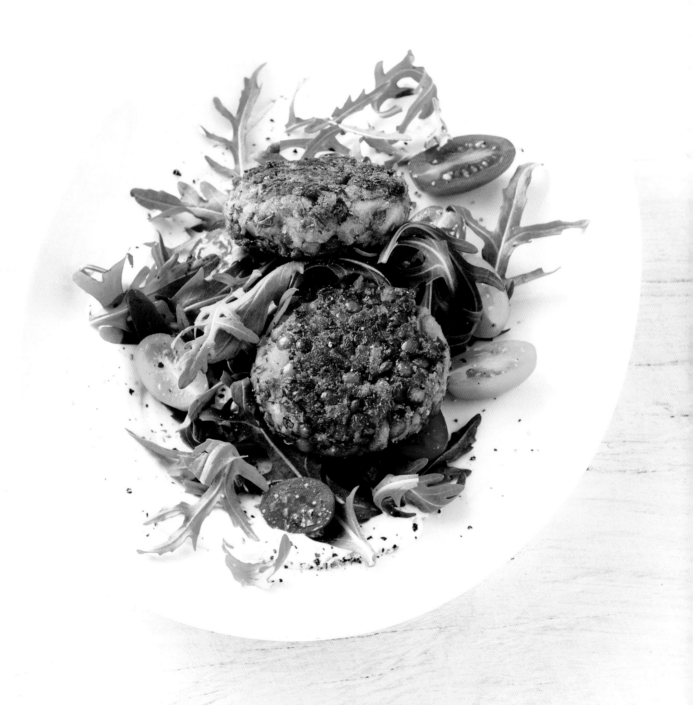

LENTILS WITH CRISPY
HALOUMI

Perfect as a light meal for a summer barbecue, the haloumi is the highlight of this lentil-packed salad.

SERVES 4 **PREP** 15 mins (+ 5 mins cooling) **COOK** 5 mins

1½ tbs extra virgin olive oil
150g haloumi, cut into 1.5cm cubes
60ml (¼ cup) fresh lemon juice
½ tsp ground cumin
400g can lentils, drained, rinsed
3 cups fresh continental
    parsley leaves
¾ cup fresh mint leaves
1 small red onion, halved, thinly sliced
250g cherry tomatoes, halved
1 tbs thinly sliced preserved
    lemon rind

1 Heat 2 tsp oil in a small frying pan over medium-high heat. Add haloumi. Cook, turning, for 4 minutes or until lightly browned. Remove from heat. Set aside to cool for 5 minutes.

2 Combine remaining oil, lemon juice and cumin in a large bowl. Season. Add lentils, haloumi, parsley, mint, onion, tomato and preserved lemon. Toss to combine. Serve immediately.

NON-FAST DAYS

Serve with 1 slice gluten-free multigrain bread per person. 93 cals per serve.

NUTRITION (PER SERVE)

CALS	FAT	SAT FAT	PROTEIN	CARBS
255	17.9g	7.6g	14.7g	11.8g

★★★★★

Even the local carnivore was full and thought this was tasty. Couldn't find preserved lemons so just went for a lot of lemon juice, salt and pepper. Definitely a keeper. **ALI128**

● VEGETARIAN   ○ VEGAN   ● GLUTEN FREE   ○ MAKE AHEAD   ○ FREEZABLE

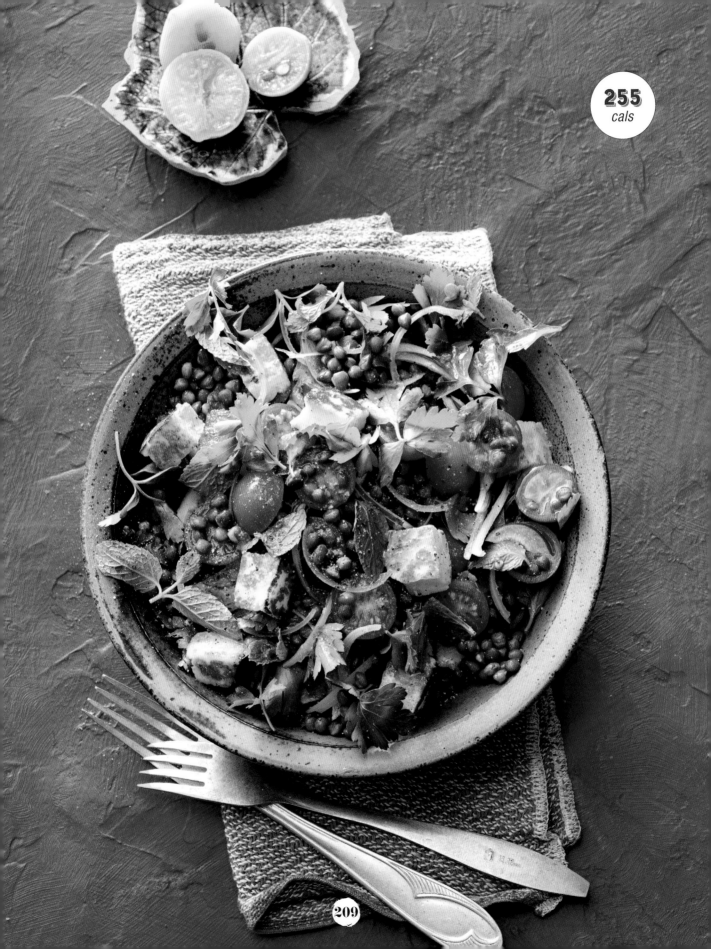

255
cals

RAINBOW SALAD JAR

This layered and colourful salad can be prepped beforehand, ready to grab on your way out the door, for a portable lunch.

SERVES 1 **PREP** 10 mins

1 tbs fresh orange juice
1 tsp olive oil
1 tsp white balsamic vinegar
½ tsp ground cumin
80g (½ cup) cooked quinoa
1 small beetroot, peeled, coarsely grated
½ zucchini, coarsely grated
1 small carrot, peeled, coarsely grated
2 tbs cottage cheese
2 tsp pepitas
Handful of mixed salad leaves

1 Combine the orange juice, olive oil, balsamic and cumin in a 500ml glass jar with a tight-fitting lid.

2 Place the quinoa in the bottom of the jar and top with beetroot, zucchini, carrot, cottage cheese, pepitas and mixed salad leaves. Cover with the lid and secure. Place in the fridge until required (up to 1 day).

3 To serve, turn into a bowl and toss to mix the layers and disperse the dressing through the salad.

NUTRITION (PER SERVE)

CALS	FAT	SAT FAT	PROTEIN	CARBS
292	10g	3g	15g	30g

NON-FAST DAYS

Add ½ cup rinsed and drained chickpeas to the quinoa. 98 cals per serve.

Nutrition tip *Aim to eat a rainbow of different vegies each day. The plant pigments in vegies are a guide to the compounds in plants that help protect our bodies against disease.* **CHRISSY FREER**

● VEGETARIAN ○ VEGAN ● GLUTEN FREE ● MAKE AHEAD ○ FREEZABLE

292
cals

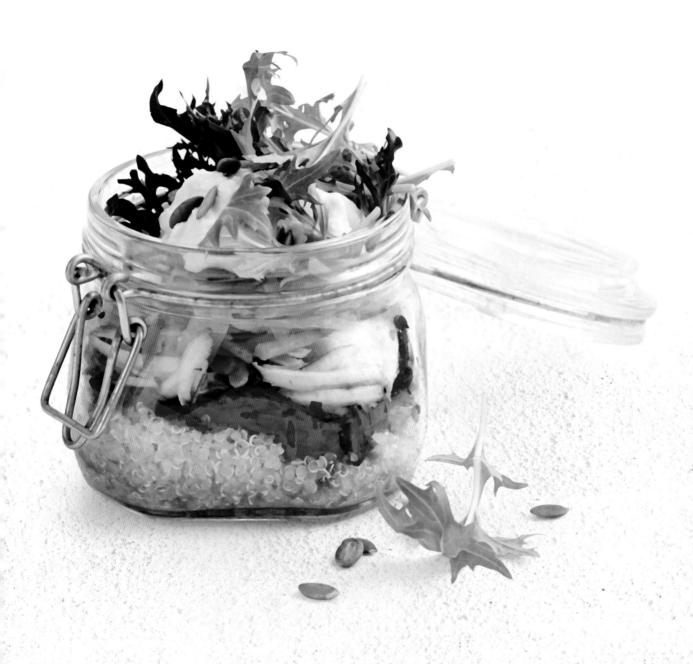

TOAST WITH HUMMUS &

EGG

Simple, yet delicious, this classic breakfast is ready in
10 minutes and has a good mix of protein, carbs and vegies.

SERVES 1 **PREP** 5 mins **COOK** 5 mins

2 small (25g each) slices seeded
  sourdough
1 tbs hummus
1 vine-ripened tomato, sliced
1 hard-boiled egg, sliced
2 tsp chopped continental parsley

1 Toast bread until golden. Spread toast with hummus.
Top with sliced tomato, egg and parsley. Season.

NUTRITION (PER SERVE)

CALS	FAT	SAT FAT	PROTEIN	CARBS
266	11g	2g	16g	23g

COOK'S NOTE

Add an extra
boiled egg for
a protein boost.
65 cals per serve.

Nutrition tip *Eggs and hummus (made from chickpeas) are both rich sources of protein. Including a serve of protein at breakfast is a great way to help you stay full throughout the morning.* **CHRISSY FREER**

● VEGETARIAN   ○ VEGAN   ○ GLUTEN FREE   ○ MAKE AHEAD   ○ FREEZABLE

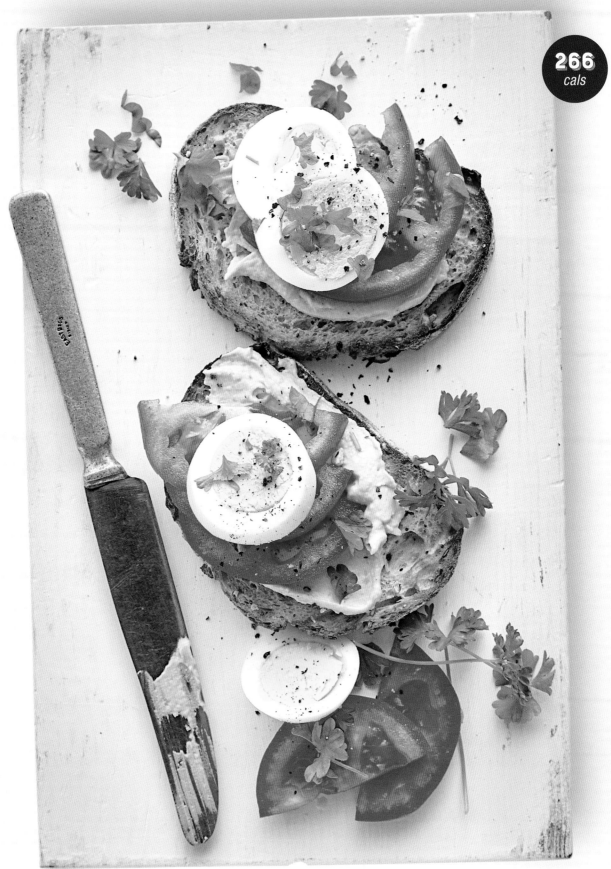

266
cals

RASPBERRY & CHIA
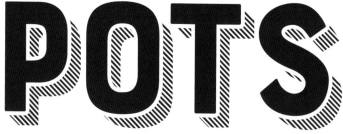
POTS

Give yourself a head start on a busy day with these pretty, but filling, make-ahead berry pots.

SERVES 2 **PREP** 5 mins (+ overnight chilling)

60g (½ cup) fresh or thawed frozen raspberries, plus ¼ cup extra, to serve
40g (¼ cup) chia seeds
25g (¼ cup) quinoa flakes
2 tsp maple syrup
185ml (¾ cup) reduced-fat milk
90g (⅓ cup) natural yoghurt, to serve

1 Place raspberries in a bowl and mash with a fork. Stir in the chia, quinoa, maple syrup and milk. Divide between 2 glasses. Cover and place in the fridge overnight to soak.
2 Top with yoghurt and sprinkle with extra raspberries. Serve in the glasses with long-handled spoon.

NUTRITION (PER SERVE)

CALS	FAT	SAT FAT	PROTEIN	CARBS
251	10g	3g	11g	22g

NON-FAST DAYS

Add 1 tbs chopped natural almonds for extra crunch. 56 cals per serve.

Nutrition tip *Raspberries are packed with dietary fibre – an impressive 8g per cup – thanks to all the tiny seeds. They're also loaded with vitamin C, are low in kilojoules and a good source of folate.* **CHRISSY FREER**

● VEGETARIAN ○ VEGAN ● GLUTEN FREE ● MAKE AHEAD ○ FREEZABLE

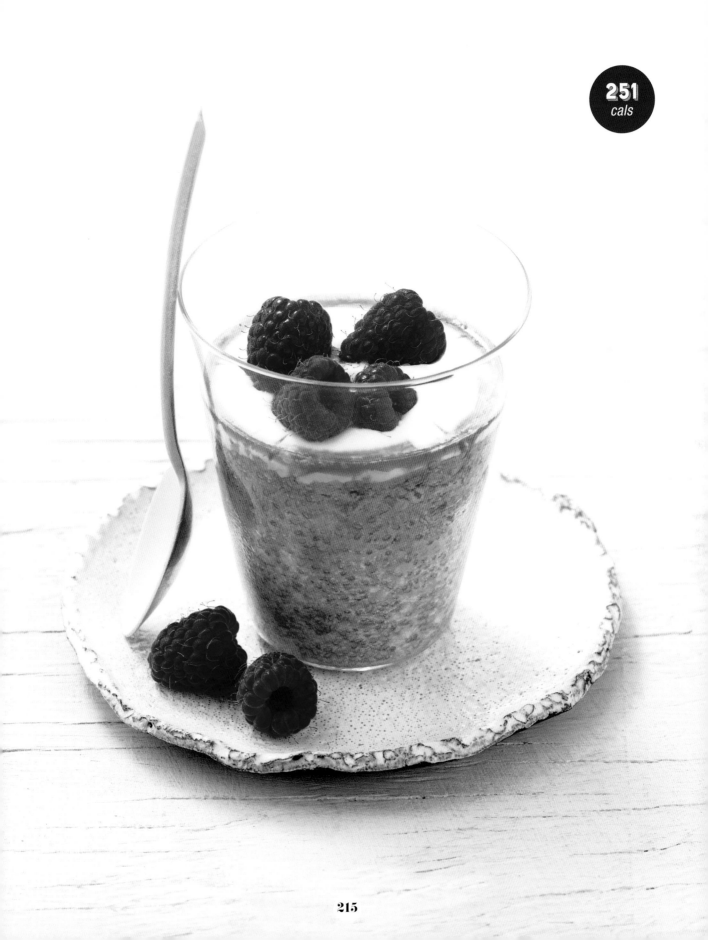

SNACKS

THESE SWEET AND SAVOURY SNACKS, ALL AROUND
125 CALORIES, WILL HELP KEEP YOU ON TRACK.

MINI TUNA & CORN FRITTATAS

These lunchbox-friendly tuna treats include plenty of essential nutrients, such as omega-3 fatty acids and vitamin D.

SERVES 16 **PREP** 10 mins (+ 5 mins standing) **COOK** 30 mins

4 eggs
80ml (⅓ cup) milk
2 tbs extra virgin olive oil
185g can tuna in springwater, drained
1 zucchini, grated
310g can corn kernels, drained
150g (1 cup) self-raising flour
85g (¾ cup) grated mozzarella
1 green shallot, thinly sliced
¼ cup coarsely chopped fresh
   continental parsley, plus extra,
   to serve

1 Preheat oven to 180°C/160°C fan forced. Grease 16 holes of two 12-hole (⅓-cup capacity) muffin pans.

2 Whisk eggs, milk and oil in a jug. Combine tuna, zucchini, corn, flour, mozzarella, shallot and parsley in a large bowl. Season. Make a well. Add milk mixture. Stir until just combined. Divide mixture among holes in prepared pans.

3 Bake for 25-30 minutes or until fritters are golden and just firm to the touch. Set aside to cool in pans for 5 minutes. Carefully transfer to a baking paper-lined wire rack to cool. Serve warm or cold, sprinkled with extra parsley.

COOK'S NOTE

Wrap frittatas individually in foil and freeze in an airtight container. Thaw at room temperature.

NUTRITION (PER SERVE)

CALS	FAT	SAT FAT	PROTEIN	CARBS
106	5.3g	1.7g	6.2g	7.9g

○ VEGETARIAN ○ VEGAN ○ GLUTEN FREE ● MAKE AHEAD ● FREEZABLE

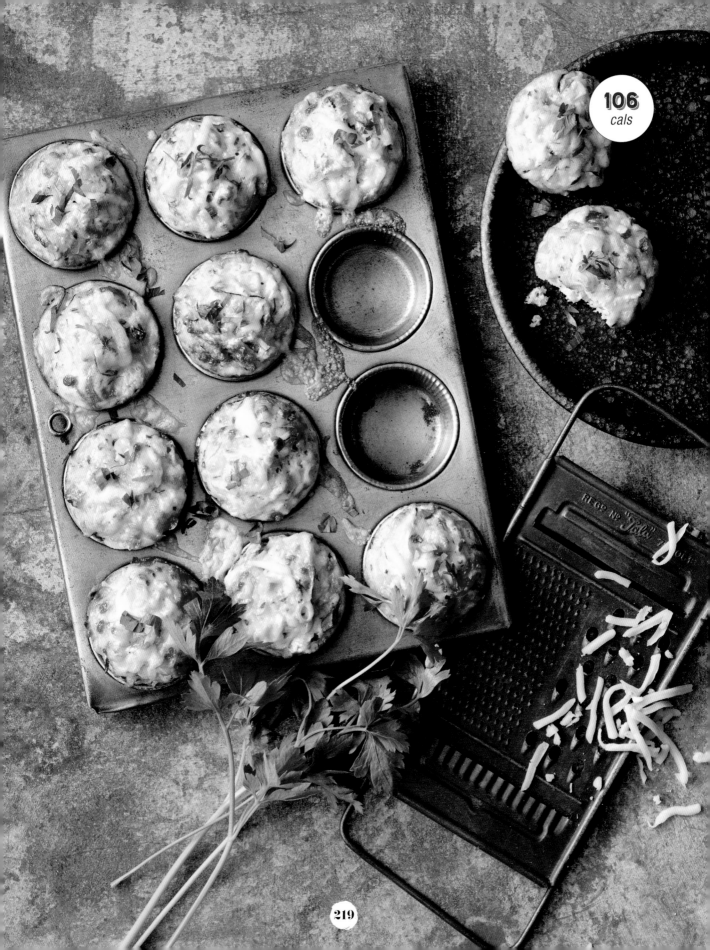

106
cals

ROASTED BEETROOT
HUMMUS

The rich colour of this dip makes it ideal for entertaining – serve with roasted vegetables for a healthy dinner party starter.

SERVES 8 **PREP** 15 mins (+ 20 mins cooling) **COOK** 50 mins

1 large (250g) beetroot, trimmed
1 tsp smoked paprika
1 tsp ground coriander
2 tsp extra virgin olive oil
400g can chickpeas, drained, rinsed
60ml (¼ cup) fresh lemon juice
2 tbs tahini
1 garlic clove, peeled, quartered
2 tbs plain Greek-style yoghurt
2 tbs fresh dill sprigs
1 tbs pine nuts, toasted
1 tbs sunflower seeds, toasted
Assorted vegetables and vegie crackers (optional), to serve

1 Preheat oven to 220°C/200°C fan forced. Wearing disposable gloves, peel beetroot. Place in the centre of a sheet of foil. Sprinkle with paprika and coriander. Drizzle with oil. Season. Fold up sides of foil to enclose beetroot, scrunching at the top to secure. Place on a small baking tray. Roast for 50 minutes or until tender. Set aside for 20 minutes to cool.

2 Transfer beetroot and spice mixture to a food processor. Process until finely chopped. Add chickpeas, lemon juice, tahini and garlic. Process until smooth and combined.

3 Transfer hummus to a serving bowl. Top with yoghurt. Season. Sprinkle with dill, pine nuts and sunflower seeds. Serve with assorted raw vegetables and vegie crackers, if you like.

COOK'S NOTE

This will keep in an airtight container in the fridge for up to 4 days.

NUTRITION (DIP ONLY, PER SERVE)

CALS	FAT	SAT FAT	PROTEIN	CARBS
122	7.7g	1.1g	4.4g	6.8g

● VEGETARIAN ○ VEGAN ● GLUTEN FREE ● MAKE AHEAD ○ FREEZABLE

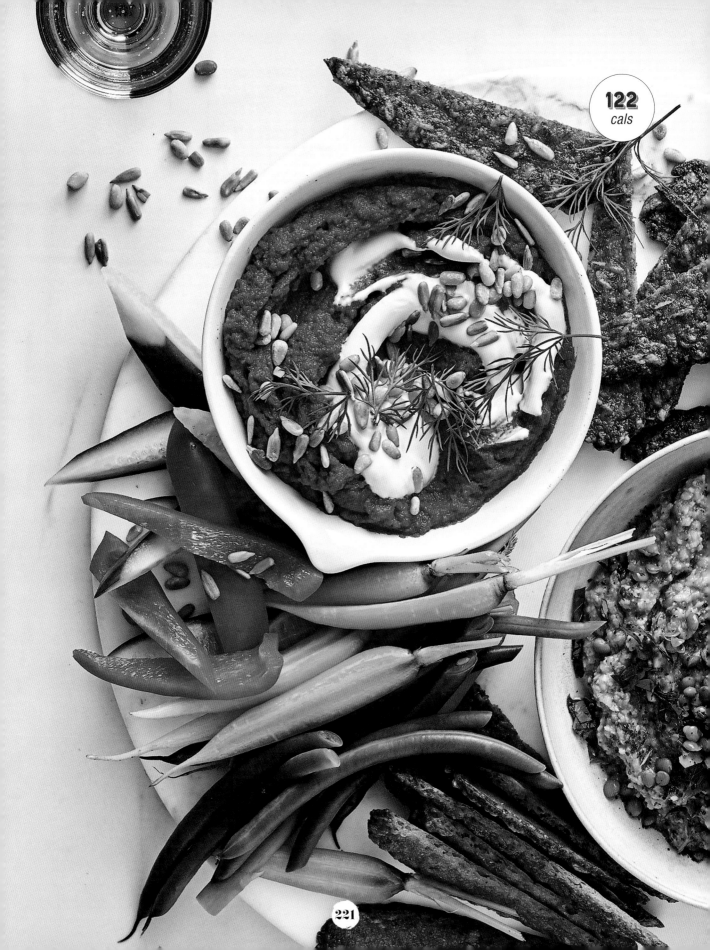

122 *cals*

SATAY BROWN RICE
BALLS

For a satisfying savoury snack, try these delicious satay balls. Lightly spiced and rolled in coconut, they are sure to become a family favourite!

MAKES 18 **PREP** 30 mins **COOK** 25 mins

200g (1 cup) brown rice
70g (⅔ cup) desiccated coconut
2 tsp coconut oil
3 green shallots, finely chopped
½ tsp turmeric
½ tsp dried chilli flakes
90g (⅓ cup) natural peanut butter
1½ tbs gluten-free soy sauce
⅓ cup fresh coriander leaves

1 Cook the rice in a large saucepan of boiling water for 25 minutes or until tender. Drain and set aside to cool.

2 Meanwhile, place the coconut in a frying pan over medium heat. Cook, stirring often, for 2-3 minutes or until light golden. Transfer to a shallow bowl and set aside to cool. Wipe frying pan clean with paper towel.

3 Heat the oil in the frying pan over medium heat. Add the shallot, turmeric and chilli flakes. Cook, stirring, for 1 minute or until aromatic. Add the peanut butter and soy sauce and stir to combine. Set aside to cool slightly.

4 Process peanut butter mixture, coriander, half the rice and ¼ cup toasted coconut until well combined. Transfer mixture to a bowl and stir in the remaining rice. Season.

5 Roll heaped tablespoonfuls of the mixture into balls. Roll balls in remaining toasted coconut to lightly coat.

COOK'S NOTE

Store rice balls in an airtight container in the fridge for up to 3 days.

NUTRITION (EACH)

CALS	FAT	SAT FAT	PROTEIN	CARBS
103	5.8g	3.2g	2.4g	9.9g

● VEGETARIAN ● VEGAN ● GLUTEN FREE ● MAKE AHEAD ○ FREEZABLE

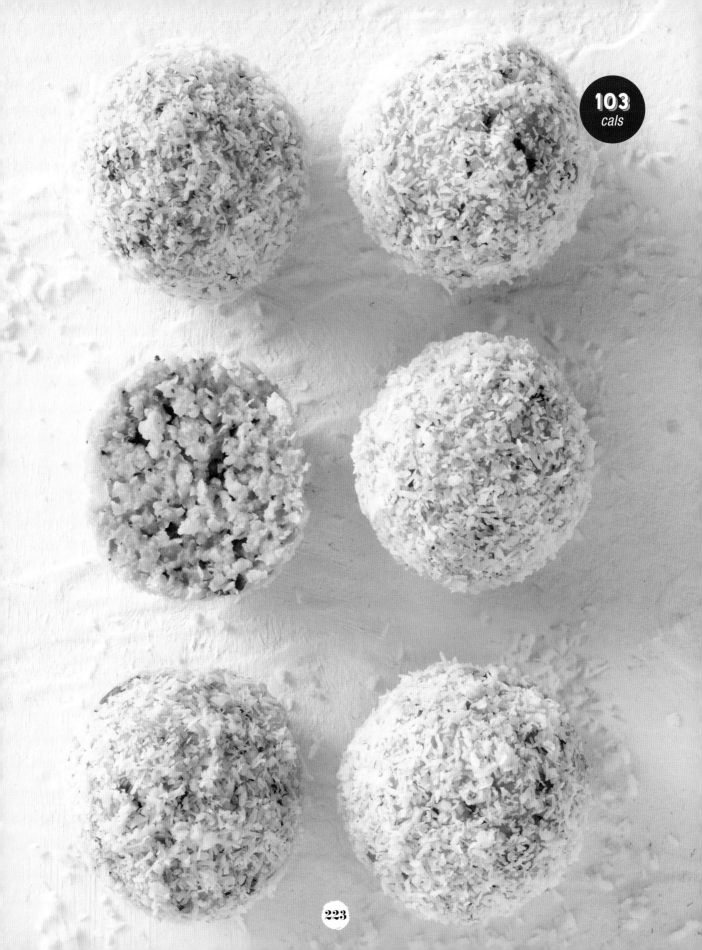

103
cals

BROAD BEAN & AVOCADO DIP

Broad beans are blended with avocado, ricotta and fresh mint to create a creamy, delicious and impressive dip.

SERVES 8 (makes 1½ cups) **PREP** 10 mins **COOK** 5 mins (+ cooling)

300g (2 cups) frozen broad beans
60g (¼ cup) smooth ricotta
20g (¼ cup) finely grated parmesan
1 avocado, coarsely chopped
2 tbs coarsely chopped fresh
   mint leaves
2 tbs fresh lemon juice
1 tsp sea salt

1 Cook broad beans following packet directions. Drain well. Peel and discard skins. Set aside to cool completely.

2 Place broad beans, ricotta, parmesan, avocado, mint leaves, lemon juice and salt in a food processor. Season with pepper. Process until smooth and combined.

COOK'S NOTE

Serve with raw vegies, such as green beans, radishes or cucumber.

NUTRITION (DIP ONLY, PER SERVE)

CALS	FAT	SAT FAT	PROTEIN	CARBS
92	7.5g	2.4g	4g	1.1g

★★★★★

This dip is really delicious. I enjoyed the refreshing tangy taste of the lemon and mint. Best avocado dip of the lot! **JACOB**

● VEGETARIAN ○ VEGAN ● GLUTEN FREE ● MAKE AHEAD ○ FREEZABLE

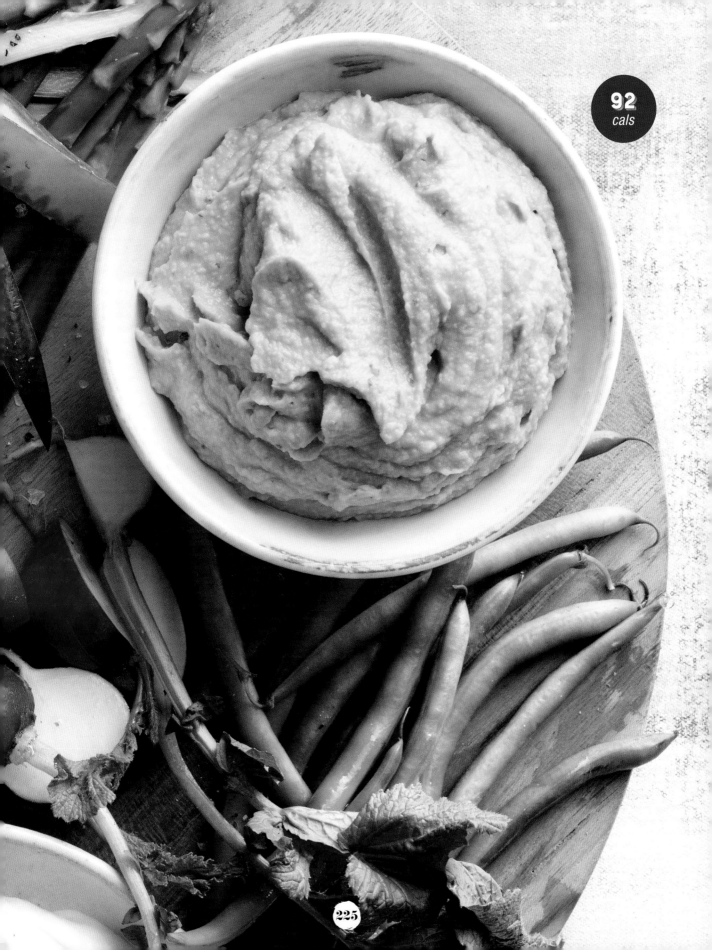

92
cals

VEGIE MUFFIN-PAN
FRITTERS

Packed full of vegies, these kid-friendly fritters are the perfect way to satisfy the after-school hungry hordes.

MAKES 12 **PREP** 20 mins (+ 5 mins cooling) **COOK** 35 mins

80ml (⅓ cup) light flavoured extra virgin olive oil
1 small zucchini, grated
1 small carrot, grated
½ cup chopped broccoli
1 tbs finely chopped fresh chives
2 tbs finely chopped fresh coriander leaves, plus extra to serve
75g (½ cup) plain flour
¼ tsp baking powder
¼ tsp sweet paprika
1 egg
60ml (¼ cup) milk
6 cherry tomatoes, halved
2 tbs sweet chilli sauce

1 Preheat oven to 220°C/200°C fan forced. Place 1 tsp oil in each hole of a 12-hole (⅓-cup capacity) muffin pan. Bake for 10 minutes or until oil is hot.

2 Meanwhile, place zucchini, carrot, broccoli, chives, coriander, flour, baking powder and paprika in a bowl. Season. Stir until well combined. Whisk egg, milk and remaining oil together in a jug. Add to vegetable mixture. Stir to combine.

3 Carefully remove pan from oven. Divide mixture among pan holes. Top with tomato halves, cut-side up. Return to oven. Bake for 20-25 minutes or until golden and crisp.

4 Brush fritters with sweet chilli sauce. Set aside in pan for 5 minutes to cool. Using a butter knife, carefully lift fritters from pan. Serve sprinkled with extra coriander.

COOK'S NOTE

Keep leftovers in the fridge for up to 2 days. Reheat in the oven.

NUTRITION (EACH)

CALS	FAT	SAT FAT	PROTEIN	CARBS
98	7g	1.1g	1.7g	6.8g

● VEGETARIAN ○ VEGAN ○ GLUTEN FREE ○ MAKE AHEAD ○ FREEZABLE

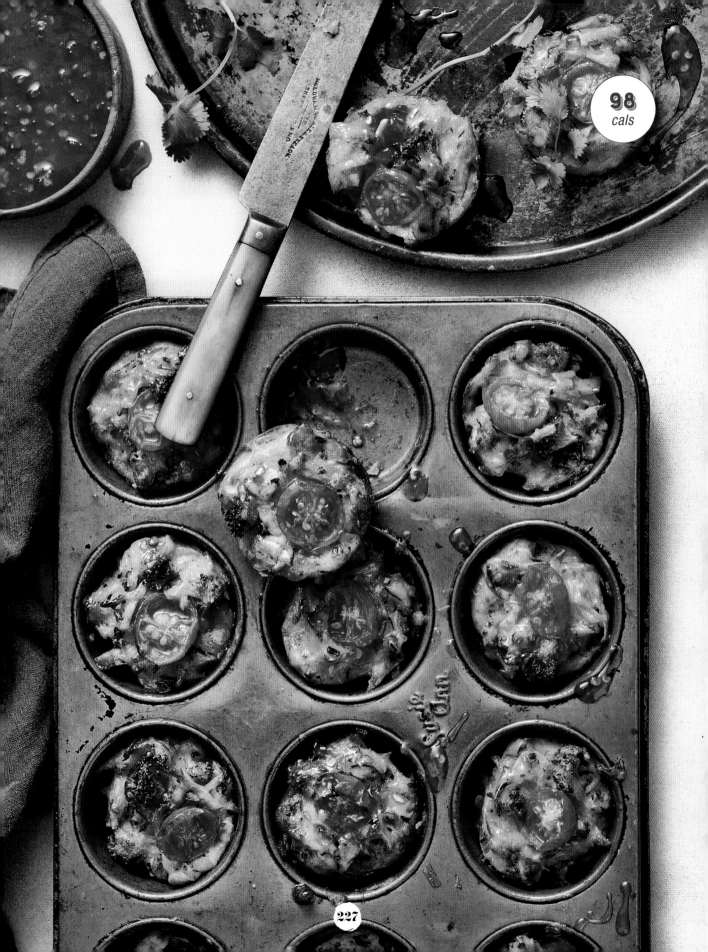

98
cals

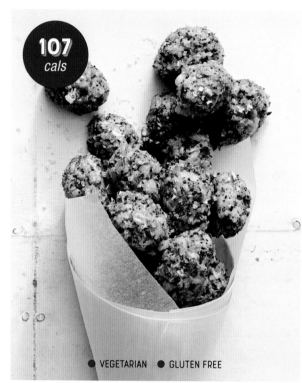

107 cals

● VEGETARIAN ● GLUTEN FREE

BROCCOLI QUINOA
NUGGETS

SERVES 6 **PREP** 15 mins **COOK** 20 mins

1 Preheat oven to 200°C/180°C fan forced. Line a large baking tray with baking paper.

2 Blanch **200g broccoli florets**. Drain and refresh under cold water. Squeeze out excess water. Place in a food processor and process until coarsely chopped. Add **½ cup quinoa flakes**, **½ cup cooked quinoa**, **60g grated haloumi**, **2 chopped green shallots** and **2 lightly beaten eggs**. Pulse to combine. Season.

3 Shape level tablespoonfuls firmly into oval shapes and place on prepared tray. Spray with oil. Bake for 15 minutes, until golden. Serve hot.

NUTRITION (PER SERVE)

CALS	FAT	SAT FAT	PROTEIN	CARBS
107	4.1g	1.6g	7.6g	2.3g

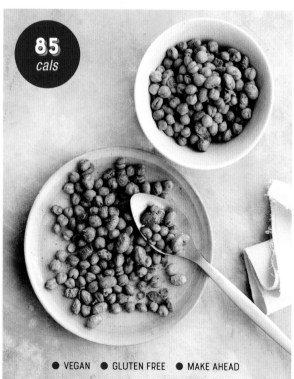

85 cals

● VEGAN ● GLUTEN FREE ● MAKE AHEAD

SPICED CHICKPEAS &
EDAMAME

SERVES 6 **PREP** 10 mins (+ cooling) **COOK** 40 mins

1 Preheat oven to 200°C/180°C fan forced. Line 2 large baking trays with baking paper. Spread **400g can chickpeas, rinsed, drained**, on a double thickness of paper towel and gently rub to remove as much moisture as possible. Repeat with **400g pkt frozen edamame, thawed, podded**. Transfer chickpeas and edamame to a large bowl.

2 Spray with oil and toss to coat. Sprinkle with **2 tsp turmeric**, **2 tsp paprika**, **2 tsp cumin** and a **pinch of cayenne pepper**. Toss to coat evenly. Transfer to prepared trays. Season with salt. Bake, tossing halfway through cooking, for 40 minutes or until well browned and crisp. Set aside on the trays to cool completely.

NUTRITION (PER SERVE)

CALS	FAT	SAT FAT	PROTEIN	CARBS
85	2.5g	0.2g	5g	8.4g

GREEN POWER
SLUSHIE

SERVES 2 **PREP** 10 mins

1 Remove and discard skin from **¼ (450g) pineapple** and coarsely chop. Place in a blender with **1 cup firmly packed baby spinach, 1 cup firmly packed fresh mint leaves, 2 tbs fresh lemon juice** and **3 cups ice cubes.** Blend until smooth.

2 Pour into two chilled 2-cup capacity glasses. Serve slushies immediately.

NUTRITION (PER SERVE)

CALS	FAT	SAT FAT	PROTEIN	CARBS
77	0.3g	0.02g	2.3g	13.2

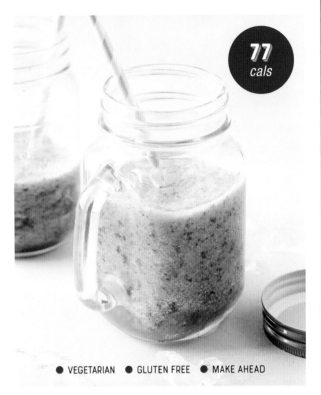

77 *cals*

● VEGETARIAN ● GLUTEN FREE ● MAKE AHEAD

CREAMY LEMON & WHITE
BEAN DIP

SERVES 8 **PREP** 5 mins

1 Drain and rinse **420g can butter beans**. Reserve 1 tbs. Place remaining beans, **½ tsp finely grated lemon rind, 1 tbs fresh lemon juice, 2 tbs extra virgin olive oil, 1 small garlic clove, crushed,** and **1½ tbs finely chopped fresh continental parsley, thyme or dill** in a food processor. Process until smooth. Season.

2 Transfer mixture to a serving bowl. Top with reserved beans. Sprinkle with **finely chopped herbs** and drizzle with **olive oil**. Serve with vegie sticks for dipping.

NUTRITION (PER SERVE)

CALS	FAT	SAT FAT	PROTEIN	CARBS
82	6g	0.8g	1.9g	3.8g

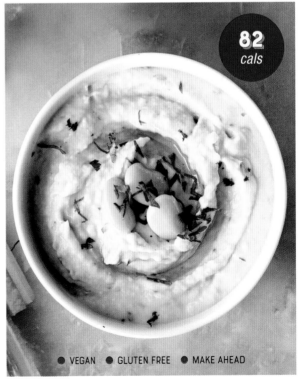

82 *cals*

● VEGAN ● GLUTEN FREE ● MAKE AHEAD

FROZEN RASPBERRY MARBLE BITES

Fruity, tangy and impressive, these pretty bites of berry and yoghurt will refresh the kids – what more can you ask?

MAKES 36 **PREP** 20 mins (+ 4 hours freezing)

10 medjool dates, pitted
50g (½ cup) instant oats
20g (¼ cup) desiccated coconut
60ml (¼ cup) melted coconut oil
200g fresh raspberries
590g (2¼ cups) Greek-style yoghurt
2 tsp white chia seeds

1 Cut 36 small strips of baking paper and use to line 30ml-capacity mini muffin pans, with ends extending above the top of the pan.

2 Process dates, oats, coconut and coconut oil in a food processor until well combined. Press 1 teaspoonful of mixture into base of each muffin hole.

3 Place raspberries in a bowl. Mash until well crushed. Add yoghurt and fold through raspberry to create a marble effect. Spoon 1 level tablespoonful of yoghurt mixture into each prepared pan. Tap pan on the bench a few times to release any air bubbles and flatten. Sprinkle with chia seeds. Freeze for 4 hours or until firm.

4 Dunk the base of the pans into warm water for 2-3 seconds, then use the paper to lift each bite out of the pan. Place in an airtight container with sheets of baking paper between layers.

COOK'S NOTE

Store bites in the freezer for up to 2 weeks.

NUTRITION (EACH)

CALS	FAT	SAT FAT	PROTEIN	CARBS
65	3.5g	0.2g	5g	8.4g

● VEGETARIAN   VEGAN   ○ GLUTEN FREE   ● MAKE AHEAD   ● FREEZABLE

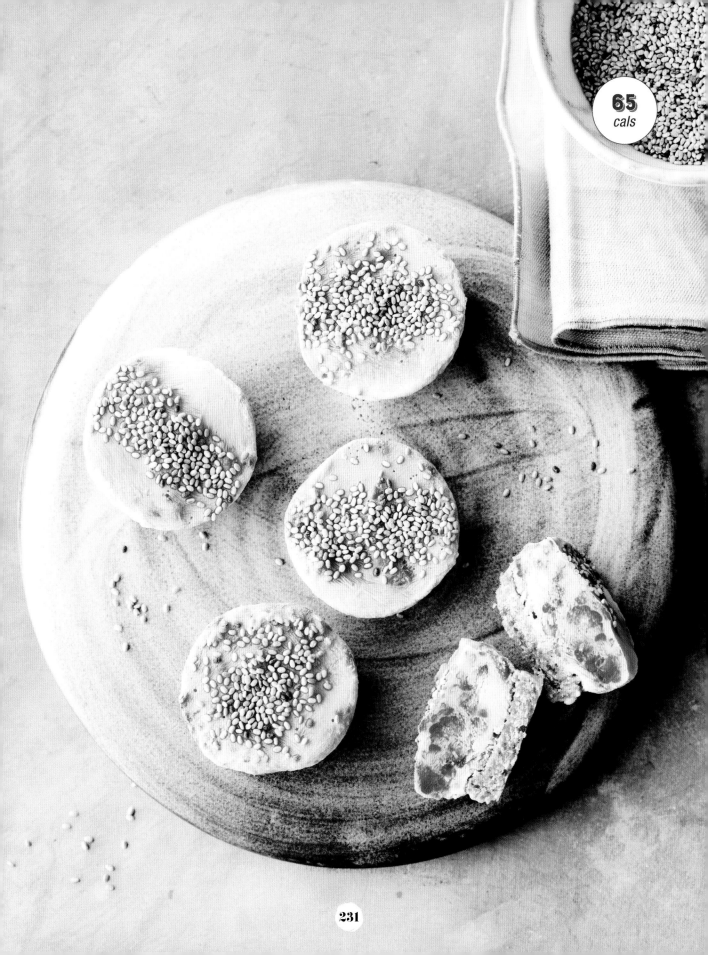

65
cals

HONEY, WALNUT & OLIVE OIL
GINGIES

Made with olive oil instead of butter, these ginger biscuits have just the right mixture of sweetness and zing.

MAKES 60 **PREP** 20 mins (+ standing & cooling) **COOK** 30 mins

340g (2¼ cups) self-raising flour
1 tbs ground ginger
1 tsp baking powder
¼ tsp bicarbonate of soda
165ml (⅔ cup) extra virgin olive oil
185ml (¾ cup) honey
2 tsp vanilla extract
1 egg, lightly beaten
2 tsp finely grated lemon rind
60g (½ cup) chopped walnuts

1 Preheat the oven to 180°C/160°C fan forced. Grease and line 3 large baking trays with baking paper.

2 Sift flour, ginger, baking powder and bicarb soda into a large bowl. Make a well in the centre. Add oil, 125ml (½ cup) honey, vanilla, egg and lemon rind. Mix well to combine. Set aside for 10 minutes to thicken slightly.

3 Roll 2 level teaspoonfuls of mixture into a ball and flatten. Press 1 side into walnuts. Place, walnut-side up, on prepared tray. Repeat with remaining mixture and walnuts. Bake, 1 tray at a time, for 10 minutes or until golden.

4 Meanwhile, combine remaining honey and 2 tbs water in a small saucepan over medium heat. Cook for 2-3 minutes or until warmed and combined. Brush honey mixture over hot gingies. Cool on trays.

COOK'S NOTE

Store in an airtight container for up to 3 days, or freeze in sealable plastic bags with all the air expelled, for up to 1 month.

NUTRITION (EACH)

CALS	FAT	SAT FAT	PROTEIN	CARBS
64	3.4g	0.4g	0.8g	7.5g

● VEGETARIAN ○ VEGAN ○ GLUTEN FREE ● MAKE AHEAD ● FREEZABLE

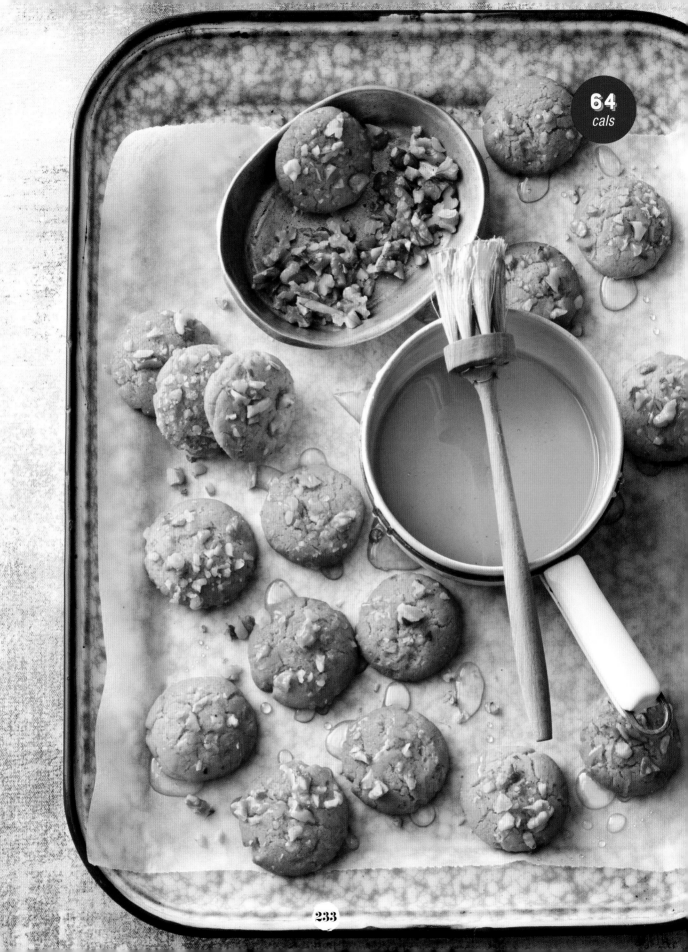

64
cals

TROPICAL COCONUT
TREATS

Sweet, yet low-cal and gluten-free, these fruity bites will hit the right spot as a midafternoon pick-me-up.

MAKES 18 **PREP** 30 mins (+ 2 hours soaking and 3 hours chilling)

150g dried sweetened pineapple
120g macadamias
1½ passionfruit, pulp removed
2 tbs coconut flour
2 tbs coconut oil
3½ tbs white chia seeds
35g (⅓ cup) desiccated coconut

1 Place the pineapple and macadamias in separate bowls. Cover with cold water. Set aside for 2 hours to soften. Drain well and pat dry with paper towel.

2 Process the pineapple and macadamias in a food processor until smooth and combined. Add the passionfruit pulp, coconut flour, coconut oil, 1½ tbs chia seeds and 2 tbs desiccated coconut. Process until the mixture comes together.

3 Spread the remaining desiccated coconut and chia on a plate. Line an airtight container with baking paper. Roll tablespoonfuls of the pineapple mixture into balls. Roll in the coconut mixture to coat. Place in the prepared container. Repeat to make 18 balls. Cover and place in the fridge for 3 hours or until just firm.

COOK'S NOTE

Store in an airtight container in the fridge for up to 5 days.

NUTRITION (EACH)

CALS	FAT	SAT FAT	PROTEIN	CARBS
105	24g	13.6g	5.8g	38.9g

● VEGETARIAN ● VEGAN ● GLUTEN FREE ● MAKE AHEAD ○ FREEZABLE

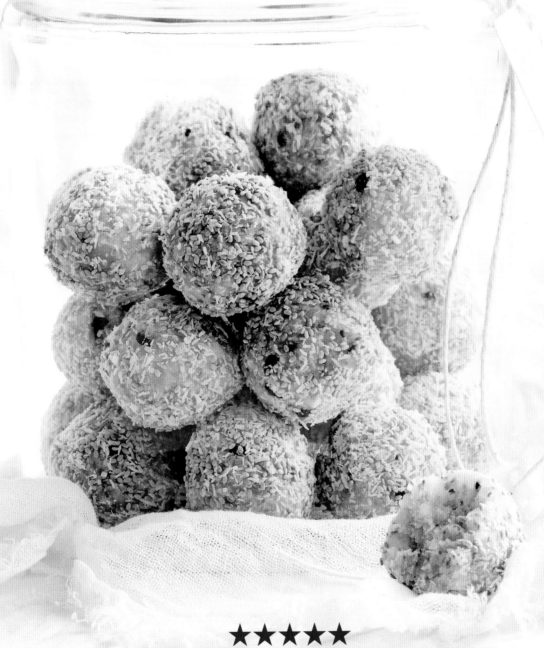

★★★★★

These are delicious! I made them as a gift for a friend who is gluten free and she now makes them once every couple of weeks. **ALYSE-GRACE**

SALTED CARAMEL & SESAME 'FUDGE'

Dates, coconut and tahini combine to create a salty and sweet (and gluten-free) treat. Maple syrup adds sweetness.

MAKES 28 cubes **PREP** 40 mins (+ 4 hours 40 mins chilling)

500g medjool dates, pitted, chopped
75g (¼ cup) hulled tahini
1 tbs coconut oil
¼ tsp sea salt, plus extra, to sprinkle
55g (⅓ cup) sesame seeds, toasted
CACAO DIP
35g (⅓ cup) raw cacao powder
75g (⅓ cup) solid coconut oil
60ml (¼ cup) maple syrup

1 Grease base and sides of a 9 x 21cm (base measurement) loaf pan and line with baking paper, allowing sides to overhang.

2 Process dates in a food processor until finely chopped. Add tahini, oil and salt. Process until well combined and smooth. Transfer to a bowl. Stir in sesame seeds. Spoon into prepared pan. Smooth surface. Place in fridge for 4 hours or until firm.

3 Line 2 baking trays with baking paper. Remove sesame mixture from pan. Use a hot, dry knife to cut into squares. Place on prepared trays and place in the fridge to cool.

4 To make the cacao dip, place all ingredients in a heatproof bowl over a saucepan of simmering water. Cook, stirring, until melted and smooth. Remove from heat. Set aside for 2 minutes to cool slightly.

5 Use 2 forks to turn caramels in cacao dip to coat. Drain off excess. Return to prepared tray. Place in fridge for 10 minutes or until set. Repeat with remaining cacao dip (reheating if necessary) to double coat, placing on remaining prepared tray. Leave until almost set. Sprinkle with a little extra salt. Place in the fridge for 30 minutes to set completely. Store in a lined airtight container in the fridge for up to 1 week.

NUTRITION (EACH)

CALS	FAT	SAT FAT	PROTEIN	CARBS
120	6g	4g	2g	14g

● VEGETARIAN ● VEGAN ● GLUTEN FREE ● MAKE AHEAD ○ FREEZABLE

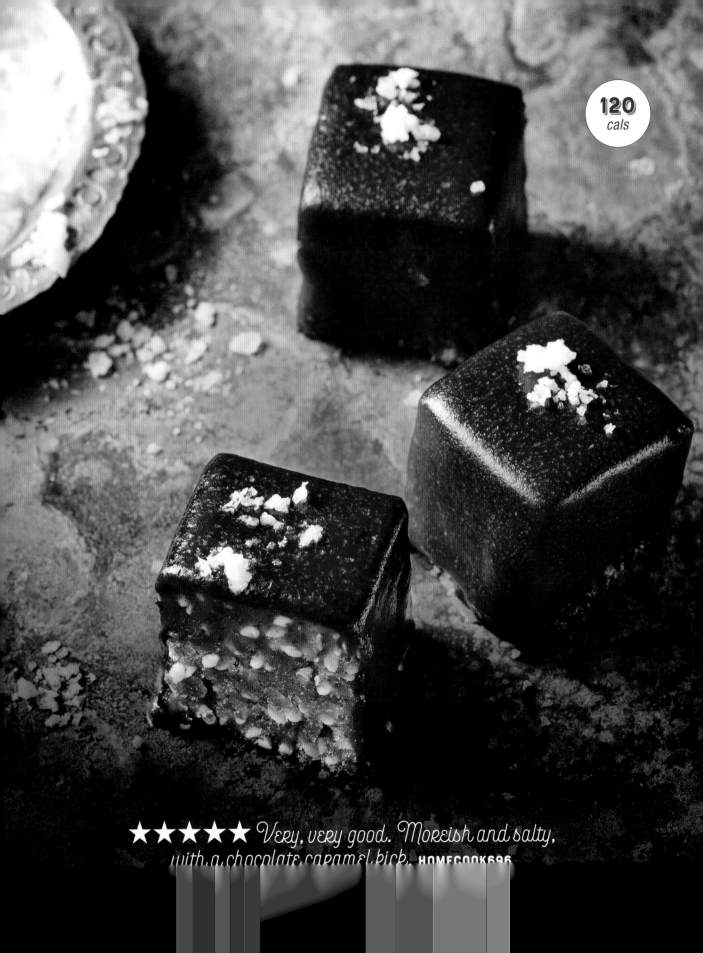

★★★★★ *Very, very good. Moreish and salty, with a chocolate caramel kick.* HOMECOOK696

MILO BLISS
BALLS

Made with coconut and rolled oats, these Milo bliss balls are the perfect on-the-go chocolatey snack.

MAKES 24   **PREP** 15 mins   **COOK** 5 mins

35g (⅓ cup) desiccated coconut
50g (½ cup) rolled oats
55g (⅓ cup) sunflower seeds
40g (¼ cup) sesame seeds
400g medjool dates, pitted
70g (½ cup) Milo, plus extra, to coat

1 Place the coconut in a small frying pan over medium heat. Cook, stirring occasionally, for 2 minutes or until lightly toasted. Transfer to a plate.

2 Wipe the frying pan clean. Add the oats, sunflower seeds and sesame seeds. Cook, stirring occasionally, for 2 minutes or until toasted. Transfer to a food processor. Set aside to cool slightly before processing until coarse crumbs form.

3 Add the dates and Milo to the food processor and process until well combined.

4 Roll 1 tbs of mixture into a ball. Repeat with the remaining mixture. Spread the extra Milo on a plate. Roll half the balls into the Milo to coat. Roll the remaining balls into the coconut to coat.

COOK'S NOTE

Store in an airtight container in the fridge for up to 1 week.

NUTRITION (EACH)

CALS	FAT	SAT FAT	PROTEIN	CARBS
87	2.4g	1.2g	1.6g	14g

● VEGETARIAN   ○ VEGAN   ○ GLUTEN FREE   ● MAKE AHEAD   ○ FREEZABLE

87 cals

★★★★★ *Super quick and easy to make. Just enough naughtiness to curb the chocolate cravings.* **STACEY_RAYMOND**

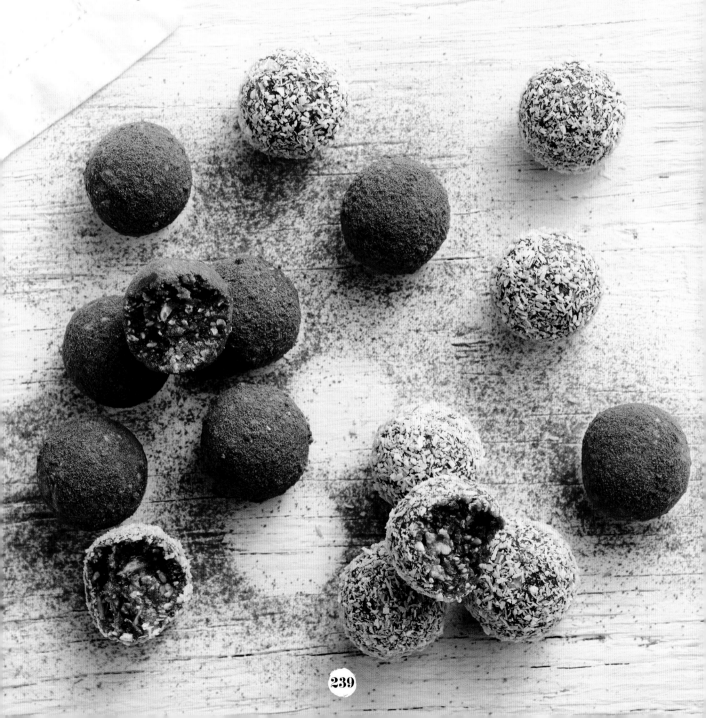

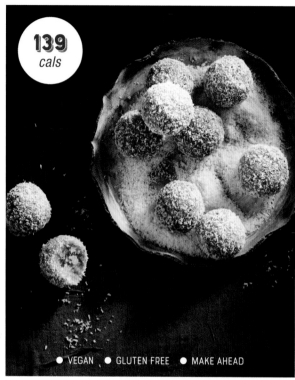

139 *cals*

● VEGAN ● GLUTEN FREE ● MAKE AHEAD

PEACH & MACADAMIA
BOMBS

MAKES 18 **PREP** 20 mins (+ 2 hours chilling)

1 Place **200g chopped dried peaches, 150g (1 cup) macadamia nuts, 2 tbs white chia seeds, 1½ tbs coconut oil, 1 tsp finely grated lemon rind** and **35g (⅓ cup) desiccated coconut** in a food processor. Process until finely chopped. Add **1 tbs fresh lemon juice** and process until a sticky mixture forms.

2 Spread another **35g (⅓ cup) desiccated coconut** on a plate. Roll level tablespoonfuls of peach mixture into balls. Roll in coconut to coat. Place in an airtight container in the fridge for 2 hours or until firm. Keep in an airtight container in the fridge for up to 1 week.

NUTRITION (EACH)

CALS	FAT	SAT FAT	PROTEIN	CARBS
139	11g	5g	2g	8g

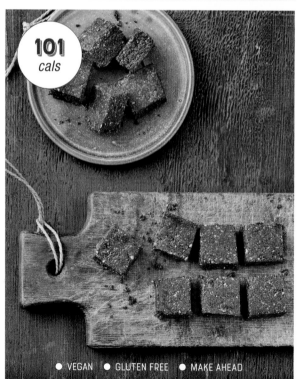

101 *cals*

● VEGAN ● GLUTEN FREE ● MAKE AHEAD

DAIRY-FREE CHOC
SLICE

MAKES 24 **PREP** 15 mins (+ overnight chilling)

1 Place **120g skinless hazelnuts** in a large frying pan over medium heat. Cook, tossing, for 3-4 minutes or until golden and toasted. Transfer to a bowl to cool completely.

2 Grease a 6cm-deep, 9 x 19cm (base measurement) loaf pan. Line with baking paper, extending paper 2cm above edges. Place **290g (1½ cups) pitted and halved medjool dates, ½ cup gluten-free almond spread,** hazelnuts, **35g (⅓ cup) gluten-free cocoa powder** and **2 tsp vanilla extract** in a food processor. Process until mixture comes together and starts to clump. Press mixture into prepared pan. Smooth top. Cover and chill overnight or until firm.

3 Remove fudge from pan and transfer to a chopping board. Cut into 24 small squares to serve.

NUTRITION (EACH)

CALS	FAT	SAT FAT	PROTEIN	CARBS
101	7g	0.7g	2.3g	7.9g

EASY STRAWBERRY
ICE-POPS

MAKES 12 **PREP** 5 mins (+ 5 hours freezing)

1 Divide **375g hulled and sliced strawberries** among **12 ice-block moulds**, pressing some of the slices against sides of each mould.

2 Pour **coconut water** into each mould to fill, leaving a 5mm gap at the top. Freeze for 1 hour or until just starting to set. Insert a wooden stick into the centre of each mould. Freeze for 4 hours or overnight.

3 To remove ice-blocks from moulds, run moulds under warm water for 10 seconds to loosen. Serve immediately.

NUTRITION (EACH)

CALS	FAT	SAT FAT	PROTEIN	CARBS
17	0.2g	0.1g	0.5g	2.9g

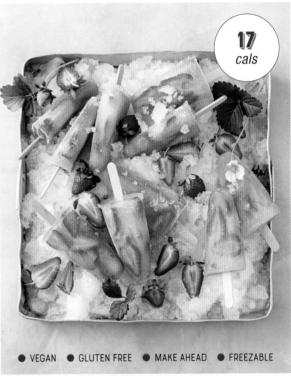

17 cals

● VEGAN ● GLUTEN FREE ● MAKE AHEAD ● FREEZABLE

BERRY GRANOLA FRO-YO
BARK

SERVES 8 **PREP** 15 mins (+ overnight freezing)

1 Grease a 20 x 30cm lamington pan. Line base and sides with baking paper, extending paper 2cm above edges.

2 Place ⅓ **cup frozen mixed berries, thawed,** in a food processor. Process until puréed. Spread **325g (1¼ cups) Greek-style yoghurt** thinly over base of pan. Dollop teaspoonfuls of berry purée over, then use a butter knife to swirl purée through yoghurt to create a marbled effect. Sprinkle with ½ **cup crispy oat clusters with strawberries.**

3 Crumble about **1 tbs freeze-dried strawberries** into a bowl to form a fine powder. Sprinkle another **1 tbs freeze-dried strawberries** over yoghurt mixture. Dust with strawberry powder. Freeze for 6 hours or overnight. Break into pieces and serve immediately.

NUTRITION (PER SERVE)

CALS	FAT	SAT FAT	PROTEIN	CARBS
92	4.8g	2.9g	2.5g	7.5g

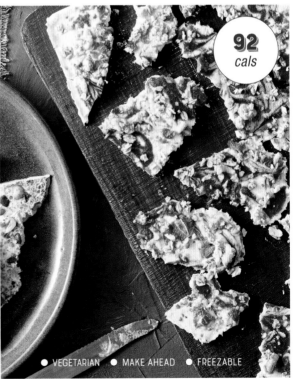

92 cals

● VEGETARIAN ● MAKE AHEAD ● FREEZABLE

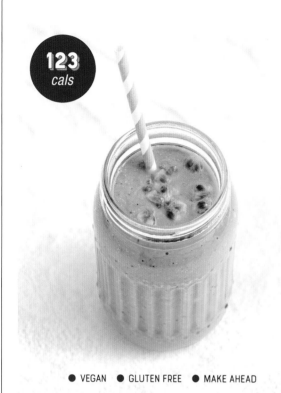

123 *cals*

TROPICAL KALE
SMOOTHIE

SERVES 1 **PREP** 5 mins

1 Combine **100g frozen mango, 20g trimmed kale, 1 tbs chopped fresh mint leaves, 250ml (1 cup) coconut water** and half the pulp of **1 passionfruit** in a blender. Blend on high speed until smooth, thick and creamy. Serve topped with remaining passionfruit pulp.

NUTRITION (PER SERVE)

CALS	FAT	SAT FAT	PROTEIN	CARBS
123	22g	4g	2.4g	52g

● VEGAN ● GLUTEN FREE ● MAKE AHEAD

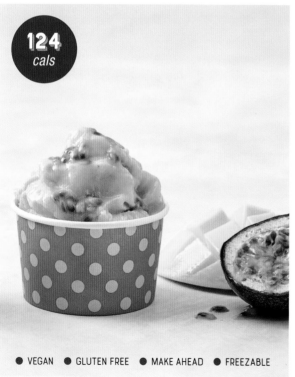

124 *cals*

PEACH & MANGO NICE
CREAM

SERVES 4 (makes 3 cups) **PREP** 25 mins (+ freezing)

1 Line a baking tray with baking paper. Cut a cross in the base of **1 yellow peach**. Place in a small heatproof bowl. Cover with boiling water. Set aside for 5 minutes. Drain. Set aside until cool enough to handle. Peel off skin and discard. Chop flesh, discarding stone. Peel and cut **2 ripe bananas** into 4cm pieces. Place peach, banana and **1 mango, chopped,** in a single layer on prepared tray. Freeze for 4 hours or overnight.

2 Place frozen fruit and **125ml (½ cup) unsweetened almond milk** in a food processor. Process, scraping down sides occasionally, until smooth and creamy.

3 Working quickly, spoon into serving dishes. Drizzle with pulp of **2 passionfruit**. Serve immediately.

NUTRITION (PER SERVE)

CALS	FAT	SAT FAT	PROTEIN	CARBS
124	1.2g	0.1g	2.3g	23.3g

● VEGAN ● GLUTEN FREE ● MAKE AHEAD ● FREEZABLE

FRESH SNACKS IN SEASON

Nutritious meals taste even better when you use the freshest produce.
This monthly guide will help you choose ingredients at their peak.

	Fruit	*Vegetables*		*Fruit*	*Vegetables*
JANUARY	apricots bananas lychees plums	cucumbers green beans tomatoes yellow squash	**JULY**	gold kiwifruit pink grapefruit pomegranates Seville oranges	potatoes pumpkins radishes rocket
FEBRUARY	blueberries kiwifruit nectarines raspberries	celery avocados snow peas sugar snap peas	**AUGUST**	blood oranges cumquats mandarins strawberries	broad beans garlic parsley silverbeet
MARCH	Golden Delicious apples guavas pears kiwifruit	carrots snake beans spinach sweet potato	**SEPTEMBER**	lemons grapefruit navel oranges strawberries	asparagus peas sugar snap peas watercress
APRIL	lemons mandarins quinces tamarillos	broccolini Brussels sprouts cauliflower chillies	**OCTOBER**	Granny Smith apples pawpaws pineapples watermelons	capsicums cucumbers lettuces zucchini flowers
MAY	apples oranges pomegranates star fruit	broccoli red cabbage leeks white onions	**NOVEMBER**	blueberries boysenberries cherries peaches	silverbeet sweet corn tomatoes witlof
JUNE	custard apples Fuji apples nashi pears navel oranges	beetroot borlotti beans celery fennel	**DECEMBER**	blackberries mangoes nectarines raspberries	butter beans chives eggplants zucchini

INDEX

OUR COMPREHENSIVE INDEX LISTS RECIPES
BY OCCASION, MEAL TYPE AND KEY GUIDE.

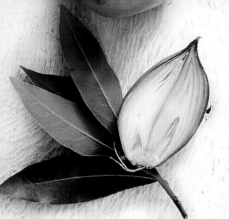
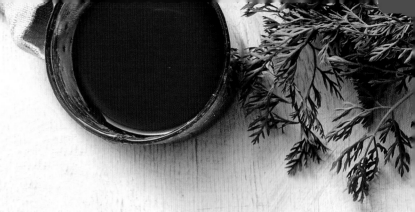

The Fast Revolution
INDEX BY OCCASION

No matter the time of day, there's a sensational
recipe here to satisfy your hunger.

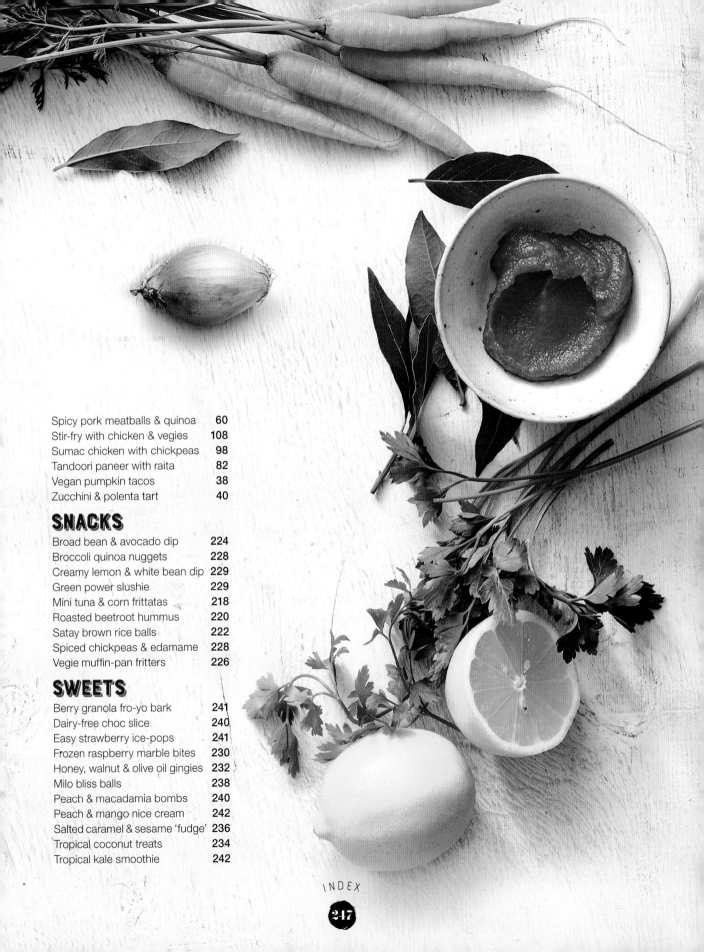

The Fast Revolution
INDEX BY MEAL TYPE

Vegetarian or omnivore, check this index for your protein preference,
to make shopping and cooking easier.

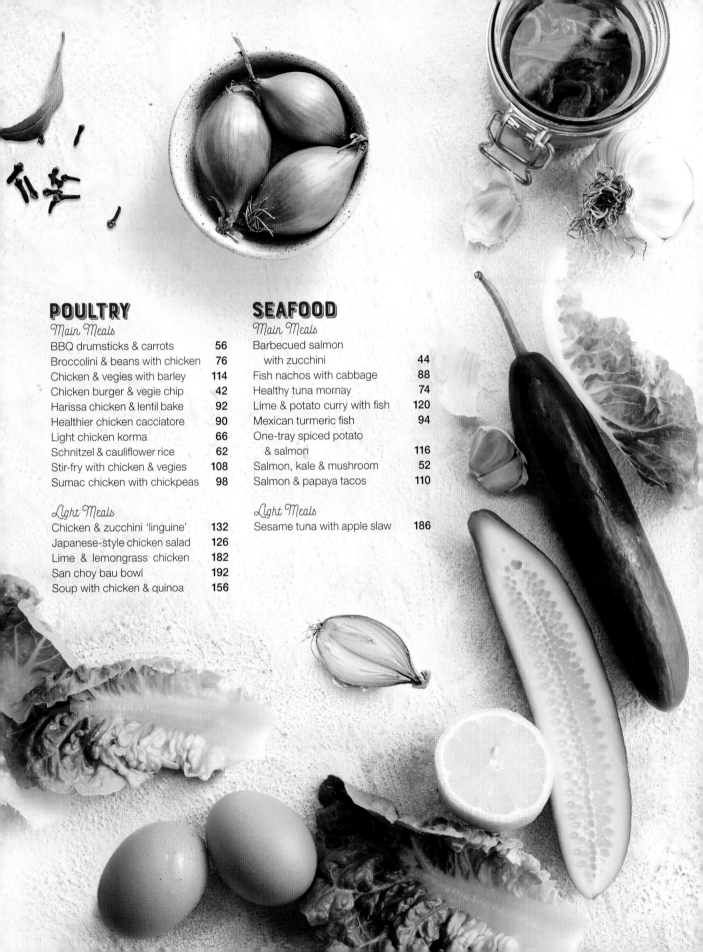

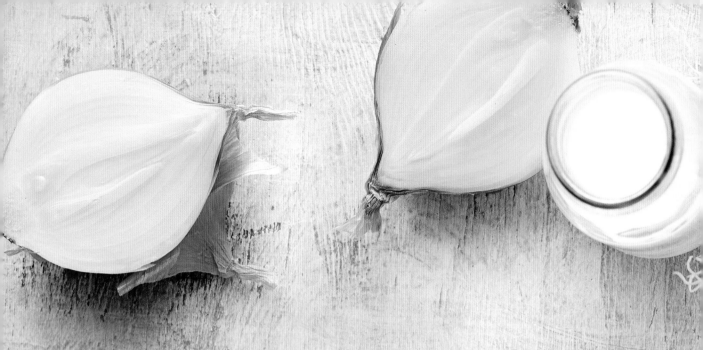

The Fast Revolution
INDEX BY KEY GUIDE

Whether you're looking for a gluten-free meal, cooking for a friend who's vegan, or just want to get organised and make ahead, we have you covered.

● VEGETARIAN

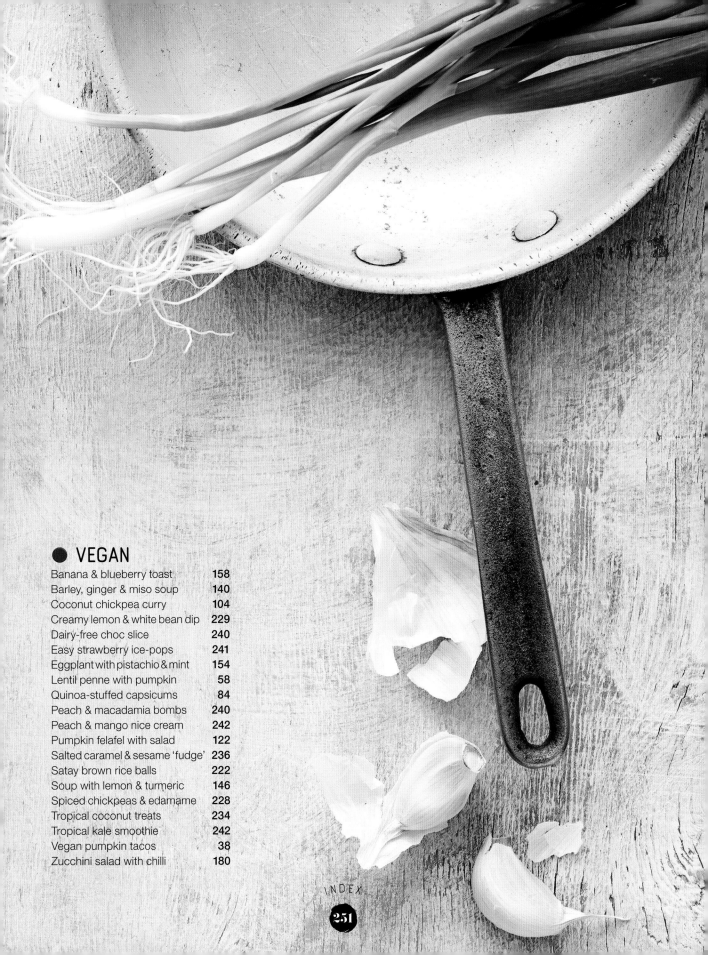

● VEGAN

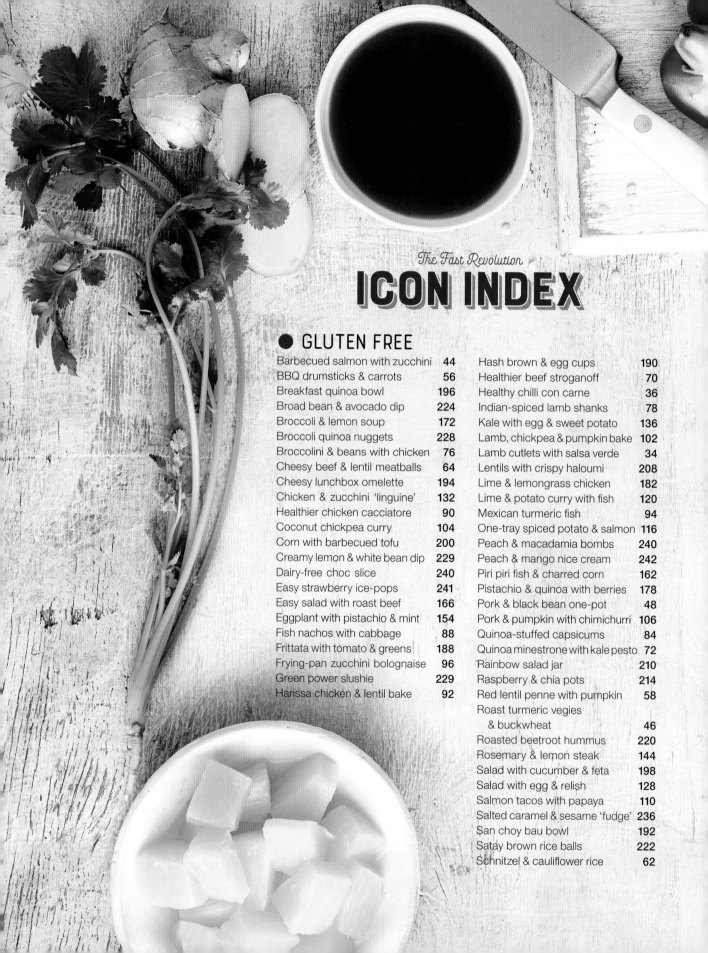

The Fast Revolution

ICON INDEX

● GLUTEN FREE

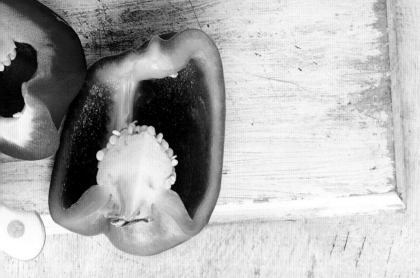
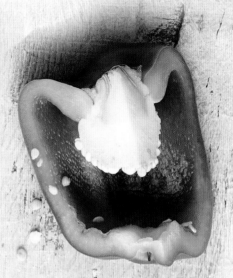

● MAKE AHEAD

● FREEZABLE

PLEASE NOTE...

While we have taken care in the preparation of this book to try to make sure the recipes and dietary labels and information are accurate, not all recipes will suit all persons living with a particular allergy or other dietary restriction. We advise anyone with food allergies or special dietary requirements to always check food labels carefully. If you think we've mislabelled a recipe, please let us know. Nothing in this book should be taken as medical or health advice.

CREDITS

editor-in-chief Brodee Myers
brodee.myerscooke@news.com.au
editor & books editor Cassie Mercer
food director Michelle Southan
book food editor Tracy Rutherford
magazine food editors Alison Adams, Miranda Payne
creative director Giota Letsios
art director Natasha Barisa
chief subeditor Alex McDivitt
subeditors Shelley Sing, Lynne Testoni, Melody Lord
design concept Rachelle Napper, Brush Media
book art director Chi Lam
nutrition editor Chrissy Freer
editorial coordinator Elizabeth Hayes

COVER IMAGES
Guy Bailey, Nigel Lough, Jeremy Simons

CONTRIBUTORS
Recipes
Alison Adams, Claire Brookman, Kim Coverdale,
Chrissy Freer, Amira Georgy, Louise Keats, Liz Macri,
Nagi Maehashi, Lucy Nunes, Kerrie Ray, Tracy Rutherford,
Michelle Southan, Katrina Woodman

Photography
Guy Bailey, Chris L Jones, Vanessa Levis, Nigel Lough,
Nagi Maehashi, Al Richardson, Jeremy Simons,
Brett Stevens, Craig Wall, Andrew Young

publishing director,
HarperCollins*Publishers* Australia Brigitta Doyle
head of Australian non-fiction,
HarperCollins*Publishers* Australia Helen Littleton

managing director, News DNA Julian Delany
director of FoodCorp Fiona Nilsson

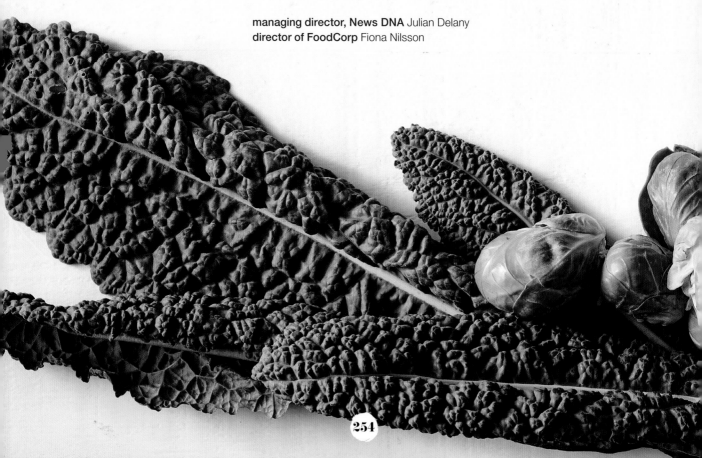

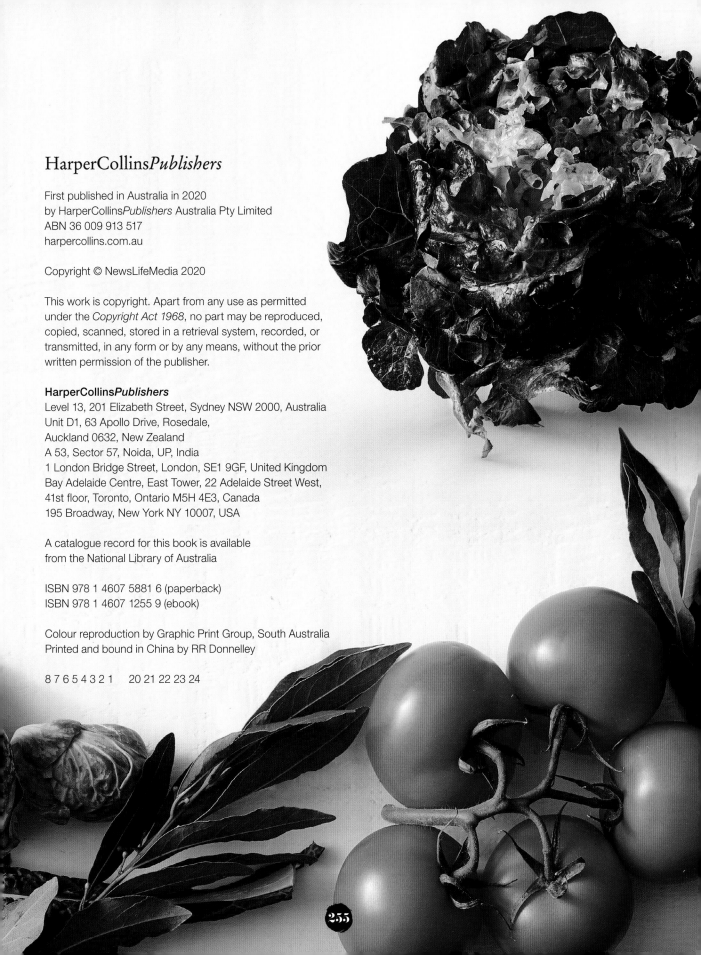

HarperCollins*Publishers*

First published in Australia in 2020
by HarperCollins*Publishers* Australia Pty Limited
ABN 36 009 913 517
harpercollins.com.au

HarperCollins*Publishers*
Level 13, 201 Elizabeth Street, Sydney NSW 2000, Australia
Unit D1, 63 Apollo Drive, Rosedale,
Auckland 0632, New Zealand
A 53, Sector 57, Noida, UP, India
1 London Bridge Street, London, SE1 9GF, United Kingdom
Bay Adelaide Centre, East Tower, 22 Adelaide Street West,
41st floor, Toronto, Ontario M5H 4E3, Canada
195 Broadway, New York NY 10007, USA

A catalogue record for this book is available
from the National Library of Australia

ISBN 978 1 4607 5881 6 (paperback)
ISBN 978 1 4607 1255 9 (ebook)

Colour reproduction by Graphic Print Group, South Australia
Printed and bound in China by RR Donnelley

8 7 6 5 4 3 2 1   20 21 22 23 24

THANK YOU

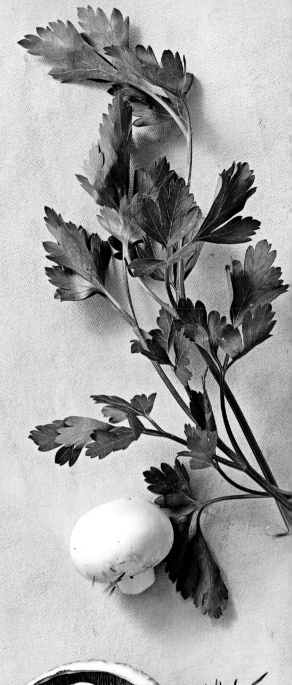

The Fast Revolution is a true collaboration by the taste.com.au team. From our stellar food team who develop the recipes, to the shoot team who make each page shine, the sub-editors who ensure each recipe is correct, and the digital team who take it to the world for everyone to cook and enjoy – each recipe is a result of amazing passion and teamwork.

A special thanks also goes to our very knowledgeable – and meticulous – nutrition editor, Chrissy Freer, for her insights and skills in helping us to bring intermittent fasting to life.

A huge thank you as well to Brigitta Doyle and Helen Littleton, our partners-in-crime at HarperCollins. You helped us bring this book alive and we're very thankful for your expertise.

We'd also like to thank... you, the audience of taste.com.au! For visiting our site every day to plan, cook and share your reviews, ratings and your recipe twists and tips. We love hearing about your passion for cooking and the gusto with which you make our recipes, so keep those reviews coming.

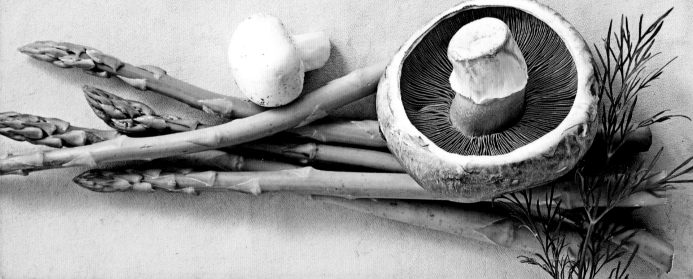